Palgrave Studies in Cyberpsychology

Series Editor
Jens Binder
Nottingham Trent University
Nottingham, UK

Palgrave Studies in Cyberpsychology aims to foster and to chart the scope of research driven by a psychological understanding of the effects of the 'new technology' that is shaping our world after the digital revolution. The series takes an inclusive approach and considers all aspects of human behaviours and experiential states in relation to digital technologies, to the Internet, and to virtual environments. As such, Cyberpsychology reaches out to several neighbouring disciplines, from Human-Computer Interaction to Media and Communication Studies. A core question underpinning the series concerns the actual psychological novelty of new technology. To what extent do we need to expand conventional theories and models to account for cyberpsychological phenomena? At which points is the ubiquitous digitisation of our everyday lives shifting the focus of research questions and research needs? Where do we see implications for our psychological functioning that are likely to outlast shortlived fashions in technology use?

More information about this series at
http://www.palgrave.com/gp/series/14636

Rachel Kowert
Editor

Video Games and Well-being

Press Start

palgrave
macmillan

Editor
Rachel Kowert
Take This
Seattle, WA, USA

Palgrave Studies in Cyberpsychology
ISBN 978-3-030-32769-9 ISBN 978-3-030-32770-5 (eBook)
https://doi.org/10.1007/978-3-030-32770-5

This Palgrave Pivot imprint is published by the registered company Springer Nature Switzerland AG
The registered company address is: Gewerbestrasse 11, 6330 Cham, Switzerland

Foreword

It's late morning on a cloudy Saturday morning and my daughter is solidly into hour two of iPad time—this morning it's *Roblox* (Roblox Corporation, 2005). I might feel guilty, but it's early and I'm tired. Also, she's got something she *really* wants me to see, and then she wants to show me the rest of her world (which usually involves wings, water, and home furnishings). Three days later, she's got out our old Nintendo DS and is playing *Animal Crossing* (Nintendo, 2001). When I come to her to tell her to get off, she stops me, saying,

"Wait, momma, do you want to see all the things I've built in the town?"

And so I take a deep breath and sit down to look over her shoulder at a bad angle and see what she's made. In five minutes she'll transition to practicing her ukulele and I'll sit on the couch playing *Alphabear 2* (Spry Fox, 2018) on my phone and listen to her awkwardly work through a new set of chords.

My daughter gets the same sense of mastery, the same creative experience, in all three of these settings. And, as this book notes, so do many, many other people. Digital games are new(ish) cousins to board games and playground games and theater games all alike, with both similar and totally new ways of providing players with a range of opportunities to develop skills, explore their inner and outer worlds, and see models for human interaction. What this book does so masterfully is to consider these models through careful parsing of the real evidence out there—instead of descending into a moral panic about screens, digital content, and online interaction.

In my work, I'm constantly talking to people who live and breathe games, and for whom digital gaming worlds are full of joy, fun, and delight. And so often, these loves exist alongside passions for gardening, or skiing, or theater, or bodybuilding.

We need good guidance, backed by good science, on how to help everyone—parents, kids, adults—understand what games can and cannot do, what they do and do not offer in terms of skill building and learning, and how they speak to and shape cultural norms and conversations. For example, in my work in the field of mental health there is fascinating early evidence about the role of games in supporting the development of skills and enabling a sense of value, achievement, and satisfaction among people with few other opportunities—not to mention the sheer joy people experience while playing.

Play has always been an essential element of human life—let's catch up to our use of it in a digital context. It is time we recognize, understand, and celebrate the ways in which games add to cultural conversations, promote play, mastery, and creativity, and help people enjoy their lives. I'm probably going to stick mostly to my cooking and yoga and backpacking, but you'll find me to be a longtime devotee of a couple of games (and a loyalist to the ones my husband makes!) and an avid watcher of the games my husband and daughter like to play.

Seattle, USA

Eve Crevoshay
Executive Director, *Take This*

References

Nintendo. (2001). *Animal Crossing* [Video game]. Nintendo Co.
Roblox Corporation. (2005). *Roblox* [Video game]. Roblox Corporation.
Spry Fox. (2018). *Alphabear 2* [Video game]. Spry Fox.

Eve Crevoshay is the executive director of Take This, whose mission is to decrease the stigma, and increase the support for, mental health in the game enthusiast community and inside the game industry. She is a 15-year veteran of the nonprofit sector, with a focus on fundraising and executing strategy. Her background spans education, social services, and the arts. She's also a yoga teacher, avid gardener and cook, and gamer. She lives in Seattle area with her husband, daughter, and two dogs.

Acknowledgements

Thank you to everyone who helped bring this project to life. Your hard work has provided a solid first step in shifting the focus away from whether or not video games *harm us* and towards how and why video games *help us* grow, learn, and thrive.

Contents

1	**Digital Games and Well-Being: An Overview** Felix Reer and Thorsten Quandt	1
2	**Press Reset** Chelsea Hughes	23
3	**Explore the Map** Shane Tilton	37
4	**Oh Me, Oh My! Identity Development Through Video Games** Sarah Sawyer	49
5	**Forever Questing and "Getting Gud"** Jamie Madigan	65
6	**Positive Psychology and Gaming: Strength and Resilience +1** Ryan Kelly	77
7	**Gaming the Mind and Minding the Game: Mindfulness and Flow in Video Games** Mark D. Cruea	97

8 Follow the Trail of Enemies 109
Emory S. Daniel Jr.

9 You Are the One Foretold; Finding Yourself Through the Journey 125
Megan Connell and Kelli Dunlap

10 Extra Lives 141
Raffael Boccamazzo

11 Concluding Comments 159
Rachel Kowert

Index 165

Notes on Contributors

Raffael Boccamazzo, Psy.D. received his doctorate in clinical psychology from the Washington State School of Professional Psychology in 2013, having completed his predoctoral internship at the Monroe Correctional Complex for the Washington State Department of Corrections. Since January 2016, he has been the clinical director of Take This—a national mental health nonprofit destigmatizing mental health challenges in the game industry. Additionally, he trains clinicians and teachers on the applied usage of role-playing games such as Dungeons & Dragons and co-founded, is an autism advocate, and is the administrator for a geek-centric psychology practice in Seattle, Washington: Save Point Behavioral Health.

Megan Connell, Psy.D. is a board-certified clinical psychologist whose practice encompasses a wide variety of topics and approaches. Her work with girls, geeks, and gamers has garnered her national attention, particularly for her work in applied role playing games such as Dungeons & Dragons. She has appeared on Geek and Sundry to talk about the interface of gaming and psychology and regularly speaks at major gaming conventions.

Mark D. Cruea, Ph.D. is an associate professor at Ohio Northern University. His research interests draw from a variety of perspectives including critical theory, political economy, reader-response theory, and feminist theory. His most recent book chapter focused on how the video game industry's business models impact the environment.

Emory S. Daniel Jr., Ph.D is an assistant professor at Appalachian State University. His research specializes in parasocial relationships/interactions, gaming, and strategic communication. His research has been published in outlets: *Journal of Interactive Advertising*, *Communication Research Reports*, *Journalism Studies*, *Internet and Higher Education Journal*, and *Journal of Advertising Education*.

Kelli Dunlap, Psy.D. is a psychologist and award-winning game designer who leverages her expertise to advocate for and advance the intersection of games and mental health. She has been recognized internationally for her work in the games and psychology space and is an outspoken advocate for mental health in and through games. Kelli earned her master's in game design from American University and her doctorate in clinical psychology from the American School of Professional Psychology. She is an adjunct faculty at the American University Game Lab and Director of Mental Health Research and Design at iThrive Games. In her spare time, she volunteers at a local animal rescue as a foster mom.

Chelsea Hughes, Ph.D. is an Insights Researcher at Riot Games. Her history of research has focused on social behavior in gaming, with specific focus on pro-social behaviors. Prior to her work in the gaming industry, she worked as a mental health practitioner specializing in college populations. She has presented about geek culture and the promotion of healthy gaming habits at universities around the world. In addition to her industry work, she frequently speaks at major gaming conventions; provides D&I education and consultation for the gaming industry; and is an award-winning cosplayer.

Ryan Kelly, Ph.D. is a clinical psychologist with a diverse practice, but with a specialty in using geek culture, tabletop games, and video games to improve therapeutic outcomes. He has published several articles and book chapters in the field of mental health and gaming. He is the co-founder of the geek-psychology media company Geeks Like Us, as well as the author and co-illustrator of *Max Gamer*, a strength-based graphic novel for Aspies. He regularly speaks at major gaming and comic conventions, institutions, and TV spots on topics like superherology, D&D and e-parenting.

Rachel Kowert, Ph.D. is the research director of *Take This*. She holds a doctorate in Psychology from the University of York (UK) and a Master of Arts in Counseling Psychology from Santa Clara University. She has published several books and scientific articles relating to the psychology of games and, more recently, the relationship between games and mental health specifically. Her most recent book, *A Parent's Guide to Video Games*, won an INDIES award in the science category.

Jamie Madigan, Ph.D. is an industrial-organizational psychologist with over 20 years of experience helping make people and workplaces better. He currently works at LeaderAmp.com as the head of product development. Dr. Madigan is also a nonfiction author and podcaster who seeks to popularize the use of psychology to understanding video games and gamified systems. He writes and podcasts at www.psychologyofgames.com and is the author of the book *Getting Gamers: The Psychology of Video Games and Their Impact on the People Who Play Them.*

Thorsten Quandt, Ph.D. is the professor of online communication at the University of Muenster, Germany. His research and teaching fields include online communication, media innovation research, digital games, and VR/AR. His work was published in leading communication and psychology journals, including Addiction, Computers in Human Behavior and Journal of Communication. He is co-editor of *The Video Game Debate*, *Multiplayer* and *Multiplayer 2*. He is the founding chair of the Digital Games Research section at the European Communication Research and Education Association (ECREA).

Felix Reer, Ph.D. is a postdoctoral researcher in the Department of Communication at the University of Muenster, Germany. His research interests include media psychology, psychosocial aspects of online communication, effects of digital games, and the use of highly immersive media technologies, such as VR and AR. He is vice-chair of the Digital Games Research Section of the European Communication Research and Education Association (ECREA).

Sarah Sawyer, Psy.D. is a licensed mental health counselor, associate clinician, and postdoctoral fellow at Sound Psychopathology and Assessment in Seattle, Washington. She specializes in integration of geek culture in the therapeutic setting, working with adults and youth, and the application of favored fictional anthologies as a therapeutic technique via role-modeling and analogous experience discussion. She has authored a clinical article for iThrive Organization, spoken on multiple academic panels, and is a moderator of the compendium library for the Geek Therapy Network.

Shane Tilton, Ph.D. is an assistant professor at Ohio Northern University. He was awarded the 2018 Young Stationers' Prize and the 2015 Outstanding New Adviser from the Society for Collegiate Journalists. His published works include the role of journalism in society and the pedagogy of gaming. His work on social media and university life earned him the BEA 2013 Harwood Dissertation Award.

List of Tables

Table 2.1	The Big 5 Personality Traits	26
Table 6.1	Relationship between subjective well-being and psychopathology	80
Table 6.2	*Dark Souls* classes and attributes	83
Table 6.3	Top rated builds from MugenMonkey character building	85
Table 6.4	Dynamic profile of strengths and weaknesses in *Dark Souls* character building	86
Table 6.5	Cloud's dynamic strengths and weaknesses profile	86
Table 6.6	Cloud's profile determined by environment	87
Table 6.7	Dynamic profile of strengths and weaknesses across diagnoses	88

CHAPTER 1

Digital Games and Well-Being: An Overview

Felix Reer and Thorsten Quandt

Abstract The public debate about digital games primarily revolves around negative outcomes of digital gaming. This bias leads to a neglect of many of the positive aspects, and in particular, digital games' contribution to well-being. However, more recently, there is a notable growth in studies interested in such beneficial effects. In this overview article, we will discuss some central research findings on three variants of well-being: hedonic, eudaimonic and social. These concepts refer to positive affective states, the fulfillment of central psychological needs and an appreciation of meaningful experiences, as well as the positive contribution to social interaction and relationships. Research on these three forms has consistently shown that games can be very effective in improving well-being.

Keywords Digital games · Hedonic well-being · Eudaimonic well-being · Social well-being · Self-Determination Theory · Meaningful entertainment

---

F. Reer (✉) · T. Quandt
Department of Communication, University of Münster, Münster, Germany
e-mail: felix.reer@uni-muenster.de

T. Quandt
e-mail: thorsten.quandt@uni-muenster.de

R. Kowert (ed.), *Video Games and Well-being*,
Palgrave Studies in Cyberpsychology,
https://doi.org/10.1007/978-3-030-32770-5_1

Since digital games entered the mass market in the 1980s, the public, as well as many scholars, have viewed them with skepticism. For example, early studies investigated whether playing video games may lead to decreases in academic performance (Harris & Williams, 1985), cardiovascular risks (Gwinup, Haw, & Elias, 1983), or epilepsy (Maeda et al., 1990). From early on, the use of violent games has been considered a possible cause of aggressiveness (e.g. Ellis, 1990); a topic that gained particular attention in the context of the school schoolings of Columbine, Erfurt, or Winnenden, and that is still being discussed controversially among scholars (Drummond, Sauer, & Garea, 2018; Scharrer, Kamau, Warren, & Zhang, 2018). Recently, the World Health Organization (WHO) decided to include the addictive use of digital games ("gaming disorder") into the International Classification of Diseases (ICD-11). This has triggered a worldwide debate about the question whether the classification in the ICD-11 is useful or not and what consequences will arise from it (e.g. Aarseth et al., 2017; Király & Demetrovics, 2017).

The dominance of research and debates on negative effects of gaming may disguise the fact that playing digital games is a very popular and entertaining spare time activity that attracts billions of players worldwide. In recent years, more and more studies on positive aspects of playing were conducted that may help to overcome the one-sided view of digital games as a risk to health and society. For example, studies examined the educational potentials of digital games in school contexts (e.g. Bai, Pan, Hirumi, & Kebritchi, 2012) or in health care and intervention (e.g. DeShazo, Harris, & Pratt, 2010). Other studies explored the benefits of using so-called exergames—a combination of digital game and physical exercise (e.g. Staiano & Clavert, 2011). Also commercial off-the-shelf games were brought in connection with positive effects, such as recovery and stress reduction (e.g. Reinecke, 2009a; Reinecke, Klatt, & Krämer, 2011).

The current chapter will overview of some of these positive effects playing digital games, with a specific focus on how the use of games may contribute to players' *well-being*. Well-being is a concept that is often associated with *positive psychology* and refers to optimal experience and sufficient mental functioning (Ryan & Deci, 2001). In particular, we will distinguish between three often-investigated subcomponents of well-being: hedonic, eudaimonic, and social well-being.

Digital Games and Hedonic Well-Being

In a general sense, the hedonic component of well-being relates to the experience of positive affective (i.e. mood) states. Hedonic understandings of well-being have often been associated with the Greek philosopher *Aristippus* who believed that living a good life in essence means maximizing individual pleasure and enjoyment and minimizing pain and suffering (Huta, 2017; Ryan & Deci, 2001). The hedonic view of well-being was also adopted by psychologists like Kahnenman and colleagues (1999) who stated that the primary aim of psychological treatment and research should be to assist people in creating pleasurable experiences and amplifying happiness as well as in reducing negative emotions like sadness or dissatisfaction (Ryan & Deci, 2001). Pleasure and happiness are two terms that have often been used to define hedonic experiences. Others include fun, enjoyment, relaxation, or carefreeness (Huta, 2017). Further, hedonic well-being was often understood as a state in absence of negative feelings, such as stress, depression, anxiety, or emotional pain (Huta, 2017).

Communication researchers and media psychologists have brought hedonic well-being in connection with the use of entertainment media, including films and television (e.g. Vorderer & Reinecke, 2012; Vorderer, Klimmt, & Ritterfeld, 2004). Viewing a comedy, reading a novel or listening to pop music can undoubtedly be pleasurable experiences that increase individual's enjoyment and well-being. A good example for a theoretical concept of entertainment research that has a clear link to the hedonic understanding of well-being is *escapism* (e.g. Katz & Foulkes, 1962). It is widely known for several decades that escaping daily life problems can be an important motivation to use media content (e.g. Hastall, 2017). From a hedonic perspective, media use thus can be seen as s sufficient strategy to (at least temporarily) increase well-being via the distraction from stress, interpersonal problems or day-to-day worries.

Concerning digital games, several studies have found that escapism and being immersed into a fantasy world to be relevant motivations of players (e.g. Scharkow, Festl, Vogelgesang, & Quandt, 2015; Sherry, Lucas, Greenberg, & Lachlan, 2006; Williams, Yee, & Caplan, 2008; Yee, 2006a, 2006b). Especially complex games like online role-playing games are often used for escapism-related motivations like immersion/fantasy (e.g. Ghuman & Griffiths, 2012; Scharkow et al., 2015). These games typically feature detailed narrations within a sophisticated virtual world and offer the fascinating opportunity to take over different identities. They thus provide an optimal environment for a pleasurable escape from the restrictions and difficulties of the real world.

While escapism is a rather broad concept that relates to many different facets of distractive media use, ***mood management theory*** (Zillmann, 1988) takes a more pronounced perspective by focusing on media-based mood regulation processes. Introduced by Zillmann (1988), mood management theory claims that the use of entertainment media can be an efficient coping strategy to bring negative mental conditions and suboptimal excitation levels back into balance (and thus to increase hedonic well-being). Studies indicate that, for example, bored individuals tend to choose exciting TV programs, while stressed individuals prefer to watch relaxing TV programs (Bryant & Zillmann, 1984). Further, participants in bad moods were found to prefer to listen to energetic-joyful music, which helped them to regulate their affective states (Knobloch & Zillmann, 2002).

In recent years, several studies have also analyzed the mood repair potentials of digital games (e.g. Bowman & Tamborini, 2012, 2015; Rieger, Frischlich, Wulf, Bente, & Kneer, 2015). For example, Bowman and Tamborini (2012) argued that digital games should be particularly well-suited to repair negative affective states since the interactivity they provide make them more demanding (and thus distracting) than non-interactive media. In a laboratory experiment with 176 participants, task demand and the participants' mood were manipulated and pre- to post-play mood repair was measured. The results indicated that higher levels of task demand (induced by varying levels of interactivity) increased the game's intervention potential and resulted in a more effective reduction of stress and boredom. In a follow-up study, Rieger et al. (2015) showed that also sadness is more effectively relieved by playing a computer game than by watching a non-interactive gameplay video.

Similarly, a survey study by Reinecke (2009a) showed that digital games are frequently used to recover from stress and strain and that work-related fatigue and daily hassles are significant predictors of the recreational use of games. Playing digital games at the workplace has also been found to have a high potential for recovery from work-related exhaustion (Reinecke, 2009b). A laboratory experiment with 160 participants showed that playing a digital game induced the highest levels of overall recovery experience in comparison to watching a non-interactive media stimulus. Further, media-based recovery experiences led to increases in vitally and cognitive performance (Reinecke et al., 2011). Taken together, these results illustrate the positive role digital games can take in increasing hedonic well-being.

Interactivity seems to be a key factor in the specific potential of games to induce hedonic well-being. The possibility to influence what happens on the screen fundamentally changes the reception process and transforms the role of the media user from a passive viewer to an active player. Becoming a famous knight in a medieval fantasy world, beating others in a shooter game, or winning the championship with one's own professional football team provide unique gratifications that other types of media can hardly offer. Unsurprisingly, achievement and experiencing success were found to be important motivations for playing digital games (e.g. Williams et al., 2006; Yee, 2006a). *Effectance* is a psychological concept that has been applied to explain the particular interactivity-based gratifications of digital games (e.g. Klimmt, 2017; Klimmt, Hartmann, & Frey, 2007).

Effectance relates to the inherently positive feeling that humans experience when interacting with the environment and realizing that their actions have an impact or make a difference (Klimmt, 2017). Small children that throw down a pencil again and again and wait for their mother to pick it up experience effectance as well as users of a computer that press a mouse button and notice a direct reaction on the screen. Digital games induce particularly strong and continuous feelings of effectance: all important events happening in a digital game are bound to the inputs of the players and only occur because the player directly caused them or at least did not prevent them (Klimmt, 2017). Further, simple commands and small inputs can have huge, direct and explicit effects on the game environment and, for example, can trigger floods, explosions, or earthquakes (Klimmt, 2017). Klimmt et al. (2007) showed that effectance experienced while playing a digital game was an important factor for the perceived game enjoyment. A deeper understanding of the link between digital game-based experiences of effectance and increases in well-being can be achieved through *flow theory* (Klimmt, 2017).

The concept of flow was established by the psychologist Csikszentmihalyi (1990) who investigated what makes people happy and under which circumstances activities contribute to life satisfaction and well-being. Flow is broadly defined as a state of optimal experience. It can arise in very different life domains and in the context of very different types of activities, such as playing chess, working, or mountain climbing (Klimmt, 2017; Sweetser & Wyeth, 2005). The most important prerequisite for the emergence of flow states is an optimal match between the skills of a person and the requirements of a task or activity (Sweetser & Wyeth, 2005). While a simple task might be experienced as boring, a too demanding task will likely lead to frustration (Klimmt, 2017). Activities that provide such an optimally balanced challenge are experienced as intrinsically motivating and lead to high levels of absorption that shift the sense of the duration of time and can offer a very pleasant relaxation from everyday life stressors (Sweetser & Wyeth, 2005).

Experiencing efficacy is a key factor contributing to the maintenance of flow states—failing in effectively manipulating the environment will immediately terminate flow (Klimmt, 2017). Digital games are particularly well-suited to enable flow: Not only do they induce strong feelings of efficacy by directly reacting to the players' inputs, but additionally offer a perfect challenge by constantly increasing in difficulty in sync with the improving skills of the user (Sweetser & Wyeth, 2005). Since regularly experiencing flow states can contribute to life satisfaction (Klimmt, 2017), playing digital games may (via its high capacity to initiate flow) not only elicit positive short-term effects, but could additionally strengthen well-being in the long run.

Taken together, there is clear evidence that the unique characteristics of digital games have a high potential to induce positive affective states as well as to resolve or relieve negative feelings. Or in other words: digital games can foster hedonic well-being. Therefore, it is not particularly surprising that digital games have already been used as tools in diverse therapeutic contexts (Griffiths, 2019). For example, digital games have already been successfully utilized in depression interventions (Li, Theng, & Schubert, 2014) and as distractors in cancer therapy and pain management (Griffiths, 2019).

Digital Games and Eudaimonic Well-Being

The term *eudaimonia* was coined by *Aristotle* who, in contrast to Aristippos and other supporters of the hedonic understanding of well-being, believed that living a good life means more than seeking for pleasure and amusement (Huta, 2017; Ryan & Deci, 2001). According to the eudaimonic understanding, real happiness is achieved through personal growth, virtuousness, and reason (Huta, 2017; Ryan & Deci, 2001). Other terms often associated with eudaimonia include meaningfulness, self-realization, autonomy, authenticity, or ethics and integration (Huta, 2017). Eudaimonic well-being is a multidimensional construct that consists of many distinct components (Wirth, Hofer, & Schramm, 2012). Several systematizations were published that help to categorize the different elements of eudaimonic well-being and to make them operationalizable for empirical research.

For example, Ryff (1989) distinguished between six different *contours* of well-being: mastery (successfully mastering the challenges of life), autonomy (experiencing self-actualization and inner freedom), personal growth (developing and expanding as a person), self-acceptance (having a positive attitude toward oneself), positive interpersonal relationships (being able to love and build up intimacy), and life purpose (finding a goal and meaning in life). According to Ryff (1989), all these elements are important factors that contribute to positive psychological functioning and well-being.

Three of the components described by Ryff (1989) also play an important role in another prominent theory that was often associated with the eudaimonic understanding of well-being: Self-Determination Theory (SDT). SDT was developed by Deci and Ryan (e.g. 2000) and assumes that human beings have three basic psychological needs and that the satisfaction of these needs is essential for well-being. The needs postulated in SDT include autonomy, competence and relatedness and, in essence, parallel Ryff's (1989) dimensions of autonomy, mastery, and positive relations. Many empirical studies have approved the assumptions of SDT: The satisfaction of autonomy, competence and relatedness needs was shown to facilitate well-being and enjoyment in a variety of contexts like, for example, the work place (e.g. Manganelli, Thibault-Landry, Forest, & Carpentier, 2018), nursing homes (e.g. Custers, Westerhof, Kuin, & Riksen-Walraven, 2010), sports teams (e.g. Quested et al., 2013), or therapy and counseling (e.g. Ryan & Deci, 2008).

In recent years, a growing number of studies have also examined in how far media use can help people to fulfill eudaimonic needs and thus can increase enjoyment and well-being (e.g. Oliver & Raney, 2011; Tamborini et al., 2011; Wirth et al., 2012). Several of these works focused on digital games (e.g. Bowman et al., 2016; Oliver et al., 2016; Ryan, Rigby, & Przybylski, 2006; Tamborini, Bowman, Eden, Grizzard, & Organ, 2010). In the following summary, we will follow Vorderer's and Reinecke's (2012) distinction between studies with a background in SDT (that investigate need satisfaction in gaming contexts) and works that are based on Beth Olivers' notion of *meaningful entertainment* (e.g. Oliver & Bartsch, 2010, 2011).

Digital Games and Psychological Need Satisfaction

In the last two decades, SDT has developed into one of the most often adopted frameworks in empirical games research. The general idea behind the application of SDT to the context of gaming is that the specific features of digital games are expected to offer a particularly fruitful ground for the satisfaction of autonomy, competence, and relatedness needs (Przybylski, Rigby, & Ryan, 2010).

First, digital games continuously confront players with new challenges and solving these tasks induces feelings of competence and mastery. The direct feedback games provide and new online technologies that allow to automatically match players based on their previous performance predestine digital games to satisfy competence needs (Przybylski et al., 2010). Second, digital games offer multiple opportunities and choices. For example, players can create their own avatars, decide what mission or level to play, and influence the future course of the happening by their in-game behaviors (Przybylski et al., 2010). The freedom of choice digital games provide can be assumed a rich source for experiences of autonomy. And third, it has become a standard that games offer multiplayer functions and possibilities to directly communicate with fellow players. Thus, games can also be considered a resource for the satisfaction of relatedness needs (Przybylski et al., 2010).

A number of empirical studies have demonstrated that digital games fulfill the basic psychological needs proposed in SDT and that need satisfaction in the gaming context contributes to enjoyment and well-being (e.g. Rieger, Wulf, Kneer, Frischlich, & Bente, 2014; Ryan et al., 2006; Tamborini et al., 2010, 2011). For example, Ryan et al. (2006) conducted three experiments using different console games and showed that playing can satisfy autonomy and competence needs. Need fulfillment, in turn, was shown to be associated with more enjoyment and pre- to post-play increases in various measures of well-being (e.g. subjective vitality, self-esteem, mood). An additional survey study among players of a multiplayer online game showed that playing together with others via the Internet can satisfy relatedness needs which was found to be associated with longer playing times and higher levels of game enjoyment (Ryan et al., 2006).

Tamborini et al. (2010) confirmed the importance of need satisfaction for game enjoyment and additionally identified several underlying factors of game-based need fulfillment, such as the physical presence of co-players (relatedness) and the perceived natural mapping of the game controls (autonomy and competence). Przybylski, Ryan and Rigby (2009) showed that also within violent first-person shooter games experiencing autonomy and competence are key factors contributing to enjoyment, while the display of violence was of minor importance for the motivation to play such games.

A more recent study by Reer and Krämer (2018) showed that joining a persistent gaming community (like a first-person shooter clan) further amplifies the potential of digital games to facilitate well-being via need satisfaction. The multiple opportunities such groups provide in terms of interacting with fellow players, improving one's game skills, participating in offline events, or helping in organizing and managing the community offer additional grounds for the satisfaction of autonomy, competence and relatedness needs (Reer & Krämer, 2018).

The potential for digital games to enhance well-being and enjoyment via the fulfillment of basic psychological needs are well documented by existing empirical studies. However, the long-term effects of game-based need satisfaction remained understudied so far. That said, it seems plausible that regularly experiencing game-based need satisfaction may also be of relevance for superordinate components of well-being, like life satisfaction or mental health.

Digital Games and Meaningfulness

The starting point of Oliver's considerations on the relationship between media use and eudaimonic well-being lay in the question why seemingly aversive media content such as dramas or tragedies are quite popular (Oliver & Raney, 2011). A merely hedonic perspective is not sufficient in explaining this phenomenon: given the negative emotions the usage can elicit (e.g. sadness, melancholia, grief), at first sight it is hard to understand how the reception of these products can be experienced as enjoyable or entertaining. According to Oliver, the use of such contents can be explained by eudaimonic motivations: people *appreciate* the *meaningfulness* of complex narrations and sophisticated media contents, even if they may also make one ruminative or even sad (Oliver & Bartsch, 2011; Oliver & Raney, 2011). In this context, *appreciation* is introduced as a eudaimonic entertainment experience that exists beyond hedonic enjoyment and is "[…] characterized by the perception of deeper meaning, the feeling of being moved, and the motivation to elaborate on thoughts and feelings […]" (Oliver & Bartsch, 2010, p. 76). It is primarily triggered by contents that have a high artistic value, that are thought-provoking and can offer new insights, or that demonstrate or teach human moral virtues (Oliver & Bartsch, 2011). In the long run, the consumption of meaningful entertainment and the experience of appreciation can "[…] strengthen individuals' general ability to confront and cope with negative experiences, thus contributing to emotional stability and eudaimonic well-being" (Bartsch & Oliver, 2017, p. 89).

Research on meaningfulness and appreciation has long focused on non-interactive media such as films. However, many digital games nowadays contain complex stories, deal with sophisticated topics, and indeed have an artistic value. Accordingly, the results of recent empirical studies have revealed that also digital games can serve as sources of meaningfulness and appreciation (e.g. Bowman et al., 2016; Oliver et al., 2016; Rogers, Woolley, Sherrick, Bowman, & Oliver, 2017).

For example, following an explorative approach, Rogers et al., asked 575 players about their most fun vs. their most meaningful video game experience. *World of Warcraft* and *Final Fantasy* were often named as meaningful games. The participants experienced games as meaningful because "[…] of a connection to characters in the game, of the story of the game, and of the moral choices allowed by the games" (Rogers et al., 2017, p. 71). In line with these findings, Bowman et al. (2016) showed that identification with a game character and feeling responsible for it are two important underlying factors of the emergence of game-based feelings of appreciation.

Oliver et al. (2016) surveyed 512 players and asked them about the game experience a fun-oriented vs. a potentially meaningful digital game provides. Meaningful games were shown to feature narrations of a higher quality than fun-oriented games. Further, they were demonstrated to satisfy the need for insight, which in turn was positively associated with experiencing appreciation (Oliver et al., 2016). A recent study by Colder Carras et al. (2018) investigated mental health benefits of gaming among military veterans and found evidence that playing did not only help the participants in terms of stress reduction, but in some cases also increased their eudaimonic well-being by offering new insights into their own situation and by giving them a new sense of self-confidence.

Even though the number of studies on the meaningfulness of digital games remains limited, there is some evidence that high quality games can induce feelings of appreciation in a similar manner as sophisticated films. Experiencing meaningfulness and satisfying needs for new insights supplements the possibilities playing provides in terms of fulfilling the three basic psychological needs postulated in SDT, thus substantially enhancing the potentials of digital games to contribute to eudaimonic well-being.

Digital Games and Social Well-Being

Undoubtedly, digital gaming has developed into a highly social activity as playing together with others (either online or offline) has come to be standard practice. According to recently published data from the American Entertainment Software Association (ESA), 56% of frequent gamers play multiplayer games at least once a week and 55% say that gaming is helpful to stay in contact with friends (ESA, 2018). The increasing possibilities for cooperative play and Internet-based communication with fellow players have made games social environments and raised the question as to whether spending time with multiplayer games may serve as a basis for the development of substantial social relationships that could increase the social embeddedness and social well-being of players (e.g. Domahidi, Festl, & Quandt, 2014; Kaye, Kowert, & Quinn, 2017; Reer & Krämer, 2019; Trepte, Reinecke, & Juechems, 2012). This question was briefly touched in the above passage on SDT and the potentials of games to satisfy relatedness needs. However, given the importance of the topic and the many existing studies that address social aspects of gaming beyond the SDT-framework, we will dedicate a separate paragraph to the possible social benefits of digital game use.

Even though first studies on social effects of gaming were already published in the 1990s (e.g. Parks & Roberts, 1998) a research boom in this area coincided with the popularization of massively multiplayer online games (MMOs) like *World of Warcraft* (Blizzard Entertainment, 2004) in the 2000s. Many of the relevant studies analyzed social effects of playing against the background of *social capital theory* (e.g. Reer & Krämer, 2014; Steinkuehler & Williams, 2006; Trepte et al., 2012; Williams, 2006a; Williams et al., 2006).

Social capital is a sociological concept that is closely linked to the works of Robert D. Putnam (e.g. Putnam, 2000). In the broadest sense, social capital can be understood as the benefits people receive from the interpersonal relationships and networks they have formed (Reer & Krämer, 2014; Trepte et al., 2012; Williams, 2006b). According to Putnam (2000), two types of social capital can be distinguished: bridging and bonding. Bridging social capital is based on informal weak ties that offer useful information, whereas bonding social capital refers to strong ties that provide emotional and material support (Reer & Krämer, 2014; Trepte et al., 2012; Williams, 2006b). Putnam (2000) demonstrated that social capital is important for many different aspects of well-being, like happiness, health, and life satisfaction.

Several studies found that MMOs and other types of online games can serve as meeting points that facilitate the formation of weak ties and bridging social capital (e.g. Steinkuehler & Williams, 2006; Trepte et al., 2012; Williams et al., 2006). For example, Williams et al. (2006) interviewed *World of Warcraft* players and found that many of them had enlarged their social networks through the game and had built casual relationships with fellow players.

Concerning the creation of bonding social capital, some early works were rather skeptical and implied that the development of deep relationships is rather seldom in gaming contexts (Steinkuehler & Williams, 2006; Williams et al., 2006). As a consequence, it was often discussed whether using online games might lead to ***displacement effects*** in the sense that meaningful offline ties are neglected in exchange for superficial gaming friendships (e.g. Kowert, Domahidi, Festl, & Quandt, 2014; Shen & Williams, 2011; Williams, 2006a). However, a recent longitudinal study did not find any signs for displacement effects (Domahidi, Breuer, Kowert, Festl, & Quandt, 2018) and other studies clearly proved that it is in general also possible for players to build up deep and meaningful relationships with fellow players (e.g. Kaye et al., 2017; Reer & Krämer, 2014, 2019; Trepte et al., 2012). The results of a study by Trepte et al. (2012) even indicated that social capital acquired in the gaming context is positively related to higher levels of offline social support. Kaye et al. (2017) recently found that game-based bonding social capital (but not bridging social capital) was associated with lower levels of perceived loneliness.

When discussing the social aspects of digital games, it is important to note that social benefits may vary strongly depending on the game, the way it is played, and the personalities and behaviors of the players. For example, playing a casual browser game may offer fewer opportunities for socializing than playing a complex online role-playing game. Even when the same game is used, players may differ in their motivations and in-game behaviors, resulting in differing social outcomes. For example, several studies have demonstrated that playing for social motivations increases the chances to experience positive social effects, while playing for escapism or achievement is less socially beneficial (e.g. Dalisay, Kushin, Yamamoto, Liu, & Skalski, 2015; Domahidi, et al., 2014; Hellström, Nilsson, Leppert, & Åslund,

2012; Reer & Krämer, 2019). Further, particular game-related behaviors such as the membership in a clan or guild, the participation in face-to-face gatherings, or the frequencies of team play and communication with fellow players were shown to foster social capital acquisition (Reer & Krämer, 2014, 2019; Trepte et al., 2012).

Concerning personality aspects, especially outgoing, extravert players were found to experience social benefits from playing (Reer & Krämer, 2017; Shen & Williams, 2011). However, this does not mean that shy, socially anxious, or introverted individuals may not also profit from playing. For example, Kowert, Domahidi, & Quandt, (2014) found that playing online games may help shy individuals to overcome their inhibitions and can support them in maintaining as well as in building up social relationships. Further, online games can serve important social functions for individuals high in attachment avoidance (Kowert & Oldmeadow, 2015). Reer and Krämer (2017) showed that at least some introverted players intentionally use online games in a compensatory manner, which enhances their chances to generate bridging as well as bonding social capital.

Taken together, there is clear empirical evidence that playing digital games in general can have positive social outcomes, which can contribute to players' well-being. However, more research is needed to deepen the understanding of the complex interplay of the many underlying factors that can influence these outcomes.

Conclusion

Digital games have been traditionally linked to negative personal and social outcomes both in the public debate and in parts of academic research: The discussed risks and effects range from inducing aggression via violent content to overuse or "addiction". Victims of these postulated negative consequences are typically adolescents and children. The reasons for this bias in the debate are manifold, but there seems to be a certain repeating pattern to portray perceived "youth" media as problematic or dangerous (as part of so-called "moral panics", see Bowman, 2016). This one-sided debate does not only characterize digital games in a misleading way—as they are far from being just youth media (Quandt, Breuer, Festl, & Scharkow, 2013)—but it also blocks the view of the beneficial effects games may have and limits the research and discussion on potential positive uses. In that sense, the negative bias in the debate may indeed have negative effects itself, by preventing a clearer understanding and exploitation of the positive aspects of digital gaming.

In this chapter, we explored the potentials of digital games on users' well-being. That is, whether digital games can contribute to a positive experience and ideal mental functioning (Ryan & Deci, 2001). As outlined above, there are three main types of well-being considered in the literature: hedonic, eudaimonic and social. In the public perception, well-being is often equated with a hedonic understanding (i.e. reaching high levels of pleasure and enjoyment paired with minimal negative feelings): People "have fun" while playing digital games, and games are used to "relieve stress" or "make gamers happy". Indeed, research on affective states has consistently shown that digital games are very effective means to positively influence the feelings of users. Gamers can escape stress or negative life-circumstances, alter or manage their mood in desired directions, experience feelings of agency and control (often in contrast to their daily life), and they consistently reach flow states that contribute to increased life satisfaction.

However, there are forms of well-being that go beyond a "(just) for fun" idea of positive affective states. Eudaimonia is a concept to describe meaningful experiences that contribute to the realization of autonomy and personal growth, and follows the idea that happiness and personal fulfillment are not just achieved by "fun" experiences. Research based on Self-Determination Theory has confirmed that digital games can serve the very basic psychological needs of their users, and by doing so, effectively contribute to enjoyment and well-being. Furthermore, there are specific types of games that seem to allow for deeply meaningful experiences via complex narrations and high artistic values. These games elicit feelings of appreciation, which in turn enhance a person's well-being.

Furthermore, digital games are not just tools to boost individual feelings of fun or meaningfulness in an isolated setting—they are often played with other humans, either co-located or online. The idea of the "lonely gamer" who plays shooter games in a darkened room without any social contact is an outdated stereotype (Kowert, Festl, & Quandt, 2014; Scharkow et al., 2015) that does not reflect the reality of most digital games users today. In addition, digital games are not only experienced in social settings—they can also be beneficial for social interactions or contribute to a person's social capital. Indeed, the respective research could highlight numerous positive effects, ranging from friendship building, overcoming inhibitions, to accumulating social capital, while debunking some of the earlier ideas that games automatically contribute to loneliness and dysfunctional relationships.

In short, games can substantially contribute to an individual's well-being, either by inducing positive affective states in various forms, by evoking feelings of appreciation for meaningful experiences, or by building social relationships and acquiring social capital. These findings need to be especially stressed in light of a rather biased discussion about the effects of digital games that seems to just focus on the negative side, and feeds a very pessimistic view.

Naturally, our call for balance in the discussion also applies to this chapter itself, and we have to admit that our overview is solely focusing on the bright side (on purpose). In all fairness, one should also mention that many of the positive potentials of games that we described in the current chapter can, under specific circumstances, also have a problematic reverse side. As we recently discussed elsewhere (Reer & Quandt, in press), the elements and mechanisms that make games enjoyable and that have the potential to strengthen hedonic, eudaimonic or social well-being were often also brought in connection with problematic, addictive forms of game use (Reer & Quandt, in press). Especially individuals with mental health challenges, those that lack meaning and need satisfaction in real life, or suffer from deficits in social integration, might find digital games so attractive that they develop excessive, unhealthy forms of engagement. This does not devaluate the positive potential of games but should never the less be kept in mind.

In many ways, games are not, by definition, "good" or "bad"—they follow the design and intentions of their producers as well as the use of the gamers. They can be a means for meaningful experiences in socially relevant settings or potentially destructive forces in the lives of some. In short: games are what we make them and how we use them. It is time that digital games start to be thought of as more than just simple entertainment but as tools to enhance our lives, including our psychological well-being.

References

Aarseth, E., Bean, A. M., Boonen, H., Colder Carras, M., Coulson, M., Das, D., … Haagsma, M. C. (2017). Scholars' open debate paper on the World Health Organization ICD-11 gaming disorder proposal. *Journal of Behavioral Addictions*, *6*(3), 267–270.

Bai, H., Pan, W., Hirumi, A., & Kebritchi, M. (2012). Assessing the effectiveness of a 3-D instructional game on improving mathematics achievement and motivation of middle school students. *British Journal of Educational Technology*, *43*(6), 993–1003.

Bartsch, A., & Oliver, M. B. (2017). Appreciation of meaningful entertainment experiences and eudaimonic well-being. In L. Reinecke & M. B. Oliver (Eds.), *The Routledge handbook of media use and well-being* (pp. 80–92). New York, NY: Routledge.

Bowman, N. D. (2016). The rise (and refinement) of moral panic. In R. Kowert & T. Quandt (Eds.), *The video game debate: Unraveling the physical, social, and psychological effects of digital games* (pp. 22–38). New York, NY: Routledge.
Bowman, N. D., & Tamborini, R. (2012). Task demand and mood repair: The intervention potential of computer games. *New Media & Society, 14*(8), 1339–1357.
Bowman, N. D., & Tamborini, R. (2015). "In the mood to game": Selective exposure and mood management processes in computer game play. *New Media & Society, 17*(3), 375–393.
Bowman, N. D., Oliver, M. B., Rogers, R., Sherrick, B., Woolley, J., & Chung, M. Y. (2016). In control or in their shoes? How character attachment differentially influences video game enjoyment and appreciation. *Journal of Gaming & Virtual Worlds, 8*(1), 83–99.
Bryant, J., & Zillmann, D. (1984). Using television to alleviate boredom and stress: Selective exposure as a function of induced excitational states. *Journal of Broadcasting & Electronic Media, 28*(1), 1–20.
Colder Carras, M., Kalbarczyk, A., Wells, K., Banks, J., Kowert, R., Gillespie, C., & Latkin, C. (2018). Connection, meaning, and distraction: A qualitative study of video game play and mental health recovery in veterans treated for mental and/or behavioral health problems. *Social Science & Medicine, 216*, 124–132.
Csikszentmihályi, M. (1990). *Flow: The psychology of optimal experience*. New York: Harper.
Custers, A. F., Westerhof, G. J., Kuin, Y., & Riksen-Walraven, M. (2010). Need fulfillment in caring relationships: Its relation with well-being of residents in somatic nursing homes. *Aging & Mental Health, 14*(6), 731–739.
Dalisay, F., Kushin, M. J., Yamamoto, M., Liu, Y.-I., & Skalski, P. (2015). Motivations for game play and the social capital and civic potential of video games. *New Media & Society, 17*(9), 1399–1417.
Deci, E. L., & Ryan, R. M. (2000). The "what" and "why" of goal pursuits: Human needs and the self-determination of behavior. *Psychological Inquiry, 11*(4), 227–268.
DeShazo, J., Harris, L., & Pratt, W. (2010). Effective intervention or child's play? A review of video games for diabetes education. *Diabetes Technology & Therapeutics, 12*(10), 815–822.
Domahidi, E., Breuer, J., Kowert, R., Festl, R., & Quandt, T. (2018). A longitudinal analysis of gaming-and non-gaming-related friendships and social support among social online game players. *Media Psychology, 21*(2), 288–307.
Domahidi, E., Festl, R., & Quandt, T. (2014). To dwell among gamers: Investigating the relationship between social online game use and gaming-related friendships. *Computers in Human Behavior, 35*, 107–115.
Drummond, A., Sauer, J. D., & Garea, S. S. (2018). The infamous relationship between violent video game use and aggression: Uncharted moderators and

small effects make it a far cry from certain. In C. Ferguson (Ed.), *Video game influences on aggression, cognition, and attention* (pp. 23–40). Cham: Springer.

Ellis, J. (1990). Computer games and aggressive behavior: A review of the literature. *Educational Technology, 30*(2), 37–40.

Entertainment Software Association (ESA). (2018). *Sales, demographic and usage data: Essential facts about the computer and video game industry*. Available at https://www.theesa.com/wp-content/uploads/2019/03/ESA_EssentialFacts_2018.pdf. Accessed June 15, 2019.

Ghuman, D., & Griffiths, M. (2012). A cross-genre study of online gaming: Player demographics, motivation for play, and social interactions among players. *International Journal of Cyber Behavior, Psychology and Learning, 2*(1), 13–29.

Griffiths, M. D. (2019). The therapeutic and health benefits of playing videogames. In A. Attrill-Smith, C. Fullwood, M. Keep, & D. J. Kuss (Eds.), *The Oxford handbook of cyberpsychology* (pp. 485–505). Oxford: Oxford University Press.

Gwinup, G., Haw, T., & Elias, A. (1983). Cardiovascular changes in video-game players: Cause for concern? *Postgraduate Medicine, 74*(6), 245–248.

Harris, M. B., & Williams, R. (1985). Video games and school performance. *Education, 105*(3), 306–309.

Hastall, M. R. (2017). Escapism. In P. Rössler (Ed.), *The international encyclopedia of media effects* (pp. 524–532). New York: Wiley.

Hellström, C., Nilsson, K. W., Leppert, J., & Åslund, C. (2012). Influences of motives to play and time spent gaming on the negative consequences of adolescent online computer gaming. *Computers in Human Behavior, 28*(4), 1379–1387.

Huta, V. (2017). An overview of hedonic and eudaimonic well-being concepts. In L. Reinecke & M. B. Oliver (Eds.), *The Routledge handbook of media use and well-being* (pp. 14–33). New York, NY: Routledge.

Kahneman, D., Diener, E., & Schwarz, N. (Eds.). (1999). *Well-being: Foundations of hedonic psychology*. New York: Russell Sage Foundation.

Katz, E., & Foulkes, D. (1962). On the use of the mass media as "escape": Clarification of a concept. *Public Opinion Quarterly, 26*(3), 377–388.

Kaye, L. K., Kowert, R., & Quinn, S. (2017). The role of social identity and online social capital on psychosocial outcomes in MMO players. *Computers in Human Behavior, 74*, 215–223.

Király, O., & Demetrovics, Z. (2017). Inclusion of gaming disorder in ICD has more advantages than disadvantages: Commentary on: Scholars' open debate paper on the World Health Organization ICD-11 gaming disorder proposal (Aarseth et al.). *Journal of Behavioral Addictions, 6*(3), 280–284.

Klimmt, C. (2017). Self-efficacy: Mediated experiences and expectations of making a difference. In L. Reinecke & M. B. Oliver (Eds.), *The Routledge handbook of media use and well-being* (pp. 157–169). New York, NY: Routledge.

Klimmt, C., Hartmann, T., & Frey, A. (2007). Effectance and control as determinants of video game enjoyment. *Cyberpsychology & Behavior, 10*(6), 845–848.

Knobloch, S., & Zillmann, D. (2002). Mood management via the digital jukebox. *Journal of Communication, 52*(2), 351–366.

Kowert, R., Domahidi, E., Festl, R., & Quandt, T. (2014). Social gaming, lonely life? The impact of digital game play on adolescents' social circles. *Computers in Human Behavior, 36*, 385–390.

Kowert, R., Domahidi, E., & Quandt, T. (2014). The relationship between online video game involvement and gaming-related friendships among emotionally sensitive individuals. *Cyberpsychology, Behavior, and Social Networking, 17*(7), 447–453.

Kowert, R., Festl, R., & Quandt, T. (2014). Unpopular, overweight, and socially inept: Reconsidering the stereotype of online gamers. *Cyberpsychology, Behavior, and Social Networking, 17*(3), 141–146.

Kowert, R., & Oldmeadow, J. A. (2015). Playing for social comfort: Online video game play as a social accommodator for the insecurely attached. *Computers in Human Behavior, 53*, 556–566.

Li, J., Theng, Y. L., & Foo, S. (2014). Game-based digital interventions for depression therapy: A systematic review and meta-analysis. *Cyberpsychology, Behavior, and Social Networking, 17*(8), 519–527.

Maeda, Y., Kurokawa, T., Sakamoto, K., Kitamoto, I., Kohji, U., & Tashima, S. (1990). Electroclinical study of video-game epilepsy. *Developmental Medicine and Child Neurology, 32*, 493–500.

Manganelli, L., Thibault-Landry, A., Forest, J., & Carpentier, J. (2018). Self-determination theory can help you generate performance and well-being in the workplace: A review of the literature. *Advances in Developing Human Resources, 20*(2), 227–240.

Oliver, M. B., & Bartsch, A. (2010). Appreciation as audience response: Exploring entertainment gratifications beyond hedonism. *Human Communication Research, 36*(1), 53–81.

Oliver, M. B., & Bartsch, A. (2011). Appreciation of entertainment: The importance of meaningfulness via virtue and wisdom. *Journal of Media Psychology, 23*(1), 29–33.

Oliver, M. B., Bowman, N. D., Woolley, J. K., Rogers, R., Sherrick, B. I., & Chung, M. Y. (2016). Video games as meaningful entertainment experiences. *Psychology of Popular Media Culture, 5*(4), 390–405.

Oliver, M. B., & Raney, A. A. (2011). Entertainment as pleasurable and meaningful: Identifying hedonic and eudaimonic motivations for entertainment consumption. *Journal of Communication, 61*(5), 984–1004.

Parks, M. R., & Roberts, L. D. (1998). Making MOOsic': The development of personal relationships on line and a comparison to their off-line counterparts. *Journal of Social and Rersonal Relationships, 15*(4), 517–537.

Przybylski, A. K., Rigby, C. S., & Ryan, R. M. (2010). A motivational model of video game engagement. *Review of General Psychology, 14*(2), 154–166.

Przybylski, A. K., Ryan, R. M., & Rigby, C. S. (2009). The motivating role of violence in video games. *Personality and Social Psychology Bulletin, 35*(2), 243–259.

Putnam, R. D. (2000). *Bowling alone: The collapse and revival of American community*. New York: Simon & Schuster.

Quandt, T., Breuer, J., Festl, R., & Scharkow, M. (2013). Digitale Spiele: Stabile Nutzung in einem dynamischen Markt. Langzeitstudie GameStat: Repräsentativbefragungen zu digitalen Spielen in Deutschland 2010 bis 2013. *Media Perspektiven, 10*, 483–492.

Quested, E., Ntoumanis, N., Viladrich, C., Haug, E., Ommundsen, Y., Van Hoye, A., … Duda, J. L. (2013). Intentions to drop-out of youth soccer: A test of the basic needs theory among European youth from five countries. *International Journal of Sport and Exercise Psychology, 11*(4), 395–407.

Reer, F., & Krämer, N. C. (2014). Underlying factors of social capital acquisition in the context of online-gaming: Comparing world of warcraft and counter-strike. *Computers in Human Behavior, 36*, 179–189.

Reer, F., & Krämer, N. C. (2017). The connection between introversion/extraversion and social capital outcomes of playing world of warcraft. *Cyberpsychology, Behavior, and Social Networking, 20*(2), 97–103.

Reer, F., & Krämer, N. C. (2018). Psychological need satisfaction and well-being in first-person shooter clans: Investigating underlying factors. *Computers in Human Behavior, 84*, 383–391.

Reer, F., & Krämer, N. C. (2019). Are online role-playing games more social than multiplayer first-person shooters? Investigating how online gamers' motivations and playing habits are related to social capital acquisition and social support. *Entertainment Computing, 29*, 1–9.

Reer, F., & Quandt, T. (in press). Entertainment theories and media addiction. In P. Vorderer & C. Klimmt (Eds.), *The Oxford handbook of entertainment theory*. Oxford: Oxford University Press.

Reinecke, L. (2009a). Games and recovery: The use of video and computer games to recuperate from stress and strain. *Journal of Media Psychology, 21*(3), 126–142.

Reinecke, L. (2009b). Games at work: The recreational use of computer games during working hours. *CyberPsychology & Behavior, 12*(4), 461–465.

Reinecke, L., Klatt, J., & Krämer, N. C. (2011). Entertaining media use and the satisfaction of recovery needs: Recovery outcomes associated with the use of interactive and noninteractive entertaining media. *Media Psychology, 14*(2), 192–215.

Rieger, D., Frischlich, L., Wulf, T., Bente, G., & Kneer, J. (2015). Eating ghosts: The underlying mechanisms of mood repair via interactive and noninteractive media. *Psychology of Popular Media Culture, 4*(2), 138–154.

Rieger, D., Wulf, T., Kneer, J., Frischlich, L., & Bente, G. (2014). The winner takes it all: The effect of in-game success and need satisfaction on mood repair and enjoyment. *Computers in Human Behavior, 39,* 281–286.

Rogers, R., Woolley, J., Sherrick, B., Bowman, N. D., & Oliver, M. B. (2017). Fun versus meaningful video game experiences: A qualitative analysis of user responses. *The Computer Games Journal, 6*(1–2), 63–79.

Ryan, R. M., & Deci, E. L. (2001). On happiness and human potentials: A review of research on hedonic and eudaimonic well-being. *Annual Review of Psychology, 52*(1), 141–166.

Ryan, R. M., & Deci, E. L. (2008). A self-determination theory approach to psychotherapy: The motivational basis for effective change. *Canadian Psychology/Psychologie Canadienne, 49*(3), 186–193.

Ryan, R. M., Rigby, C. S., & Przybylski, A. (2006). The motivational pull of video games: A self-determination theory approach. *Motivation and Emotion, 30*(4), 344–360.

Ryff, C. D. (1989). Happiness is everything, or is it? Explorations on the meaning of psychological well-being. *Journal of Personality and Social Psychology, 57*(6), 1069–1081.

Scharkow, M., Festl, R., Vogelgesang, J., & Quandt, T. (2015). Beyond the "core-gamer": Genre preferences and gratifications in computer games. *Computers in Human Behavior, 44,* 293–298.

Scharrer, E., Kamau, G., Warren, S., & Zhang, C. (2018). Violent video games do contribute to aggression. In C. Ferguson (Ed.), *Video game influences on aggression, cognition, and attention* (pp. 5–21). Cham: Springer.

Shen, C., & Williams, D. (2011). Unpacking time online: Connecting internet and massively multiplayer online game use with psychosocial well-being. *Communication Research, 38*(1), 123–149.

Sherry, J. L., Lucas, K., Greenberg, B., & Lachlan, K. (2006). Video game uses and gratifications as predictors of use and game preference. In P. Vorderer & J. Bryant (Eds.), *Playing computer games: Motives, responses, and consequences* (pp. 213–224). Mahwah, NJ: Lawrence Erlbaum.

Staiano, A. E., & Calvert, S. L. (2011). Exergames for physical education courses: Physical, social, and cognitive benefits. *Child Development Perspectives, 5*(2), 93–98.

Steinkuehler, C. A., & Williams, D. (2006). Where everybody knows your (screen) name: Online games as "third places". *Journal of Computer-Mediated Communication, 11*(4), 885–909.

Sweetser, P., & Wyeth, P. (2005). GameFlow: A model for evaluating player enjoyment in games. *Computers in Entertainment, 3*(3), article 3a.

Tamborini, R., Bowman, N. D., Eden, A., Grizzard, M., & Organ, A. (2010). Defining media enjoyment as the satisfaction of intrinsic needs. *Journal of Communication, 60*(4), 758–777.

Tamborini, R., Grizzard, M., Bowman, N. D., Reinecke, L., Lewis, R. J., & Eden, A. (2011). Media enjoyment as need satisfaction: The contribution of hedonic and nonhedonic needs. *Journal of Communication, 61*(6), 1025–1042.

Trepte, S., Reinecke, L., & Juechems, K. (2012). The social side of gaming: How playing online computer games creates online and offline social support. *Computers in Human Behavior, 28*(3), 832–839.

Vorderer, P., Klimmt, C., & Ritterfeld, U. (2004). Enjoyment: At the heart of media entertainment. *Communication Theory, 14*(4), 388–408.

Vorderer, P., & Reinecke, L. (2012). Zwei Prozess Modelle des Unterhaltungserlebens: Unterhaltung im Schnittbereich hedonischer und non-hedonischer Bedürfnisbefriedigung. In L. Reinecke & S. Trepte (Eds.), *Unterhaltung in neuen Medien. Perspektiven zur Rezeption und Wirkung von Online-Medien und interaktiven Unterhaltungsformaten* (pp. 12–29). Köln: von Halem.

Williams, D. (2006a). Groups and goblins: The social and civic impact of an online game. *Journal of Broadcasting & Electronic Media, 50*(4), 651–670.

Williams, D. (2006b). On and off the' net: Scales for social capital in an online era. *Journal of Computer-Mediated Communication, 11*(2), 593–628.

Williams, D., Ducheneaut, N., Xiong, L., Zhang, Y., Yee, N., & Nickell, E. (2006). From tree house to barracks: The social life of guilds in world of warcraft. *Games and Culture, 1*(4), 338–361.

Williams, D., Yee, N., & Caplan, S. E. (2008). Who plays, how much, and why? Debunking the stereotypical gamer profile. *Journal of Computer-Mediated Communication, 13*(4), 993–1018.

Wirth, W., Hofer, M., & Schramm, H. (2012). Beyond pleasure: Exploring the eudaimonic entertainment experience. *Human Communication Research, 38*(4), 406–428.

Yee, N. (2006a). The demographics, motivations, and derived experiences of users of massively multi-user online graphical environments. *Presence: Teleoperators and Virtual Environments, 15*(3), 309–329.

Yee, N. (2006b). Motivations for play in online games. *CyberPsychology & Behavior, 9*(6), 772–775.

Zillmann, D. (1988). Mood management through communication choices. *American Behavioral Scientist, 31*(3), 327–340.

CHAPTER 2

Press Reset

Chelsea Hughes

Abstract Anyone who has ever played a video game has likely experienced the joys of a reset button. The game didn't go well, and so you gave yourself an opportunity to do it over again. Of course, a real-life reset button doesn't exist because time is linear—what is done is done and can never be truly erased. However, that does not mean that what is done cannot be *done over* (like redoing a level to get the rest of the missing coins). There is a common misbelief our personality is unchangeable. Namely, how we were born and what we have been through firmly dictate how we are able to live our lives. Through established psychological theories and illustrative examples, this chapter will explore how our personality is not something set in stone. Rather, gaming can be used to overcome the behavioral barriers we experience in our personalities to accomplish lasting, meaningful change.

Keywords Video games · Well-being · Personality · Goal setting · Behavior

C. Hughes (✉)
Riot Games, Los Angeles, CA, USA

R. Kowert (ed.), *Video Games and Well-being*,
Palgrave Studies in Cyberpsychology,
https://doi.org/10.1007/978-3-030-32770-5_2

We all make choices, but in the end the choices make us.
—Andrew Ryan, BioShock (2K Games)

Anyone who has ever played a video game has likely experienced the joys of a reset button. The game didn't go well, and so you gave yourself an opportunity to do it over again. Perhaps you've even considered what life might be like if you had a real-life reset button:

> Got that pesky, anxious brain? *Boop! Reset.*
> Had some painful emotional experiences that you can't get past? *Boop! Start over.*
> Feel like you missed out on some key lessons for how to adult? *Boop! Let's try that again.*

Of course, a real-life reset button doesn't exist because time is linear—what is done is done and can never be truly erased. However, that does not mean that what is done cannot be *done over* (like redoing a level to get the rest of the missing coins).

There is a common misbelief our personality is unchangeable. Namely, how we were born and what we have been through firmly dictate how we are able to live our lives. Through established psychological theories and illustrative examples, this chapter will explore how our personality is not something set in stone. Rather, their mutability is the key to overcoming barriers and experiencing meaningful change by pressing reset on our lives.

What Is Personality?

If you do an Internet search on the definition of the word "personality," you are likely to get as many definitions as you have links to click. Personality is something psychologists have debated for centuries. Generally speaking, personality can be thought of as "a *social construct* that refers to *behaviors* that are *socially relevant, enduring*, and that are assumed to reflect certain *motivational properties*" (Harwood, Beutler, & Groth-Marnat, 2011). This quote highlights the core features of personality.

First, Personality Is a Socially-Relevant, Social Construct

While this may seem like semantics, it is an important note to make. Personality itself is not tangible, definite, or concrete. It is a word psychologists created to describe a pattern of behaviors that objectively seem to be related. Hundreds of theories of personality have developed over millennia, each with their own merits and reflecting the social constructs of their time.

One of the earliest documented theories of personality came from the Greek philosopher Hippocrates, around 400 BC. Hippocrates argued that there were four primary types of temperament which were dictated by varying amounts of fluids in a person's body (Jackson, 2001). These fluids, known as "humors," were central to the Greeks' understanding of medicine and human health. Culturally embedded theories of personality didn't stop then and there: constellations, horoscopes, zodiacs, moon signs, Myers-Briggs typology—these are all theories rooted in their respective cultural beliefs. The various sociocultural origins of different personality theories have one undeniable result: when people measure "personality," they are not always measuring the same thing in the same way.

Second, Personality Reflects Motivational Properties

Personality is not something that occurs at random; it serves a function and reflects our innermost workings as humans. According to Interpersonal Theory of Personality Development (Burgoon, Stern, & Dillman, 1995), everything we learn is adaptive. The tendencies we develop all serve a purpose. Typically, as children, our behaviors are driven by the desire to achieve feelings of love, safety, and comfort. These things are *good*. They feel like rewards to us. As such, any behaviors that elicit loving and caring behaviors from others are reinforced.

We've all heard the example of the mother and her child in the grocery store, right?

A mother and her child go into the checkout line at the grocery store. The child sees candy and asks for some. When the mother says no, the child starts to cry. The child, it seems, won't stop crying until their mother gives in. Things devolve into a tantrum. Finally, exhausted and defeated, the mother gives in after several minutes. In this situation, the child has learned something important: *if I want to get candy, I should throw a fit. Better yet, Mom saying "no" once or twice doesn't matter. If I* keep *throwing a fit, she'll eventually give in.*

Unfortunately for the rest of us, these learnings tend to get generalized. After several instances like the one in the grocery store, this child may grow up to discover that tantrums are the best way to get more than just candy. If they want love, safety, and comfort, they'll just throw a fit. This behavior will then become so ingrained, so enduring, so characteristic of the person, that it becomes a core aspect of their personality.

That said, it all starts with a need—to feel loved, safe, and comfortable. It's the same thing everyone wants (however that looks for them). We all learn different ways to achieve those feelings. Some learn to throw tantrums. Some learn to take care of others. Some learn to make friends, and others learn that they can only trust themselves. Ultimately, it all comes down to what we have learned about how to get our needs met.

Third, Personality Is an Enduring Pattern of Behaviors

To illustrate this point, let's focus on the most widely accepted and researched theories of personality: The Big 5 (originally formulated by Tupes & Christal, 1961). According to this theory, we can categorize the infinite and overwhelming number of human traits into five super-traits (Mount, Barrick, Scullen, & Rounds, 2005; Zillig, Hemenover, & Dienstbier, 2002), captured by the acronym OCEAN (or CANOE, if that floats your boat; see Table 2.1).

The Big 5 theory of personality suggests that most of the "essence" of a person can be accounted for by each of these five traits. For example, someone who is described as a "people-pleaser" is someone who would score high in Agreeableness and Neuroticism. A party planner who is very good at their job would probably score high in Conscientiousness and Extraversion.

Table 2.1 The Big 5 Personality Traits[a]

	Personality trait	*Defining features*
O	Openness to experience	Imaginativeness and intellectuality
C	Conscientiousness	Dependability and meticulousness
E	Extraversion	Sociability and social energy
A	Agreeableness	Cooperativeness and consideration
N	Neuroticism	Emotionality and insecurity

[a]Mount, Barrick, Scullen, and Rounds (2005)

As you look at these traits, you may notice that they are all, at least partly, defined by behaviors. Imagination is the conscious choice to pursue alternative thoughts (Vygotsky, 2004). Conscientiousness is the choice to align with goals and delay gratification (Roberts, Jackson, Fayard, Edmonds, & Meints, 2009). However, even someone who fully embodies one of these traits can practice doing the opposite. For example, an agreeable person can refuse to cooperate, and a neurotic person can learn to manage their emotions.

While these traits may seem to be rigid and unchanging at first glance, they are actually just patterns of behaviors. And like all behaviors, we have agency in learning them, enacting them, and unlearning them. It's just a matter of dedication and practice.

Putting the "U" in Username: How "You" Come Through in Gaming

For years, personality was observed formally only through traits and behaviors observable in the "real" world. Yet according to the Entertainment Software Association, 60% of American play video games daily. Moreover, 63% of American gamers play with others, and those frequent gamers average 7 hours per week playing with other people online, and 6 hours with other people in-person (ESA, 2018, 2019). In short, people spend considerable time interacting with each other in video games. Therefore, researchers have spent the past several years looking toward personality's manifestation in the online realm.

Research generally suggests that our real-world traits and behaviors are reflected in our in-game behavior. In other words, the "real-life" you maps on pretty well to the "in-game" you.

In a survey of over one thousand *World of Warcraft* players, researchers collected self-reported measures of personality and automated behavioral data reports provided by *Blizzard* (Yee, Ducheneaut, Nelson, & Likarish 2011). They used the Big 5 framework to test their theory. Across every domain, they found similarities in the players' "real-world" personality and their in-game behaviors:

- Players high in extroversion preferred group activities over solo activities in the game.

- Players high in agreeableness were more likely to send positive emotes (e.g., hugs, cheers, and waves) to other players.
- Players high in conscientiousness tended to have higher ratings in disciplined tasks, like having high cooking and fishing scores, and collecting vanity pets.
- Players high in Openness to Experience showed in-game behavioral patterns consistent with curiosity and exploration, like having more characters, more characters in more realms, and more time spent exploring.
- Players low in Neuroticism show behaviors consistent with security and emotional stability, like having characters of a different gender.

While there is a clear connection between Big 5 super-traits and in-game behaviors, we also see this reflection in more complex traits. For example, a 2016 study by Tang and Fox found that male gamers high in social dominance and hostile sexism were more likely to harass female gamers. A 2017 study by Hughes and colleagues found that social dominance predicted active social behavior in multiplayer online video games.

What does this all mean? When we play video games, we generally approach tasks and interactions the same way we would in the "real-world." Knowing this, we can adapt what we know about change and achievement within video games to achieve change and achievement in our out-of-game lives.

Hitting the Grind: Lots of Small Tasks Lead to Big Loot

I'm just a worrisome person. I always think of the worst case scenario. My dad's the same way.

With what's happened to me, I'm so suspicious of everyone. I always assume people will hurt me.

I'm a logical person. I don't really get *emotions. It makes it hard for me to connect with people, but emotional stuff doesn't click for me.*

Any of these look familiar? Unfortunately, self-beliefs that assume immutability stifle growth and become barriers to the lives we want to lead. The person with anxiety can't drive on the freeway. The person with a traumatic history can't trust people. The person who struggles with emotions can't develop meaningful connections with others.

In my years as a therapist, I heard talk like that more often than not: *It's just the way I am.* My clients saw their tendencies and believed that they were bound to them. And who could blame them? It's all they'd ever known about themselves. They had never been forced to question these things as *learned behaviors*, and therefore *un*learnable—at least, until they found themselves in my office.

The truth is that the vast majority of personal characteristics, made up of patterns of behavior and thought, are almost *always* changeable (Damian, Spengler, Sutu, & Roberts, 2018). You just have to be patient, trust in the principles of learning, and *stick to it.* Persist. Persevere (something we gamers have a lot of experience doing! For more on this, check out Chapter 4 of this book).

The first step is to conceptualize these changes as a goal you are trying to reach. According to goal-setting theory (Locke & Latham, 1990), effective goals are clear, challenging, appropriately complex (as opposed to vague or too easily achievable) and measurable. An example of an effective goal would be, "*Within 6 months, I want to stop negative self-talk, such as calling myself stupid.*" This is an effective goal because it has clear success criteria and does not require a lot of other things to fall into place. This is in contrast to an ineffective goal, such as "*I want to have healthier self-esteem.*" The success criteria for this goal is far too vague, there is no set deadline, and involves too many non-defined moving parts (i.e., how does one achieve healthier self-esteem? What is even considered "healthier"?). It may seem nitpicky, but developing skills in how to set and plan for goals is important. Proper goal-setting (even when the goals aren't achieved) been linked to subjective well-being, and has been shown to have widespread effects (MacLeod, Coates, & Hetherton, 2008).

Of course, setting the goal is just one of many steps required to actually attain any long-term change. Yet every moment, every decision, and every day provides a new opportunity to press reset and change course. How so? Rather than going into the deep science of neuropsychology and cognitive development, allow me to share with you a metaphor I frequented with my clients: *Imagine that you're trying to get through a dungeon. First thing's first, you need to ask yourself: What's at the exit? What am I going to achieve by getting through this dungeon?*

Making changes is hard, and it's even harder if you don't know why you're making those changes. It's helpful to have a goal in mind. There is no "right" goal to have. Maybe your dream armor is dropped in the final chamber of that dungeon. Maybe you just want to prove that you're capable of clearing dungeons. At the end of the day, it just needs to be *yours*, and something you're willing to stick by.

Now, you've established the goal of clearing this dungeon. It's time to find a way to make it to the end. Naturally, you look for a path—something that's been trodden before, to make the journey easier. There's one path you see: dozens of others are on it, it's super easy to follow, and you don't immediately see anything that's trying to kill you. So, you start to make your way.

As you travel along this path, you start to notice some problems with it. It twists and turns. You see familiar things, find no new monster camps, and it feels like you've been there before. (Maybe you cleared it already?) And as you continue on, it occurs to you: maybe this path doesn't lead to the end of the dungeon after all. Maybe it leads to some other chamber, or perhaps it *used to* lead to the end before the game got updated. But right now, this path is not going to get you to your final chamber. So, you turn back and start over at the beginning.

A little worn out but still determined, you look for another path. After a little bit of searching, you find one. It's a little more rugged than the path before. There are some critters trying to kill you, and it's a little hard to see, but it's still very much doable with a torch. So, you take it. Before long, you notice this path has its own problems. It might lead to the end—but it seems to have been made for a different class than you. It requires necromancy, and you're a druid (or whatever). Had you taken a different path in life, this route may have suited you just fine—and it's super frustrating to see all those Necromancers strolling along with their fancy new loot. But right now, this path is not yours to take. So, you turn back. You start over again.

Again and again, you try to find paths through this dungeon. You try to make it to your goal. Again and again, the paths don't lead you there. At this point, you probably start to ask yourself, "Is this final chamber worth it?" or "Am I worthy enough to get out of this dungeon?"

That's when you notice the explosives in your inventory.

You realize that if those previously trodden paths aren't going to get you through, you're going to have to make a path yourself. A *new* path. Right here, right now. And so, you start blowing things up.

For those of you who have never tried it, exploding your way through a stone dungeon is hard work. It takes dedication and perseverance. No single explosion is going to get you out of there. You just have to do it, again and again, until you're out. And you do! You smash a hole, kill the goblin camp, and smash another hole. Because you know, without a doubt, that blasting a hole in one direction, over and over again, is *going* to get you out of that dungeon.

> Spoiler Alert: I'm not actually talking about dungeons. The human brain works in a similar way.

Think about every thought process, every trait you have as a path through a dungeon: your extroversion, your neuroticism, your tendency to jump to a worst-case scenario. The most well-trodden path is the easiest to follow. It's already lit up for you, most of the monsters have been cleared, and it's super easy to find. Heck, there might even be some shopkeepers set up in there to reinforce the idea that you're on the right track. In fact, if you zoned out for a minute, you'd likely end up taking that path again. You're just used it.

Trying to develop a new thought is like blasting a hole through a dungeon wall. You have to actively turn away from the path and decide, in that moment, to do something different. It's hard work. Trying to develop a new *pattern of thoughts* is like blasting a hundred holes through a hundred dungeon walls, persistently and consistently. You're forging your own path, blast by blast. This work is even harder. Every goblin camp, every stone wall is a signal for you to turn back to the path you know. But with perseverance, those holes will become a path. And with dedication, that path will become *the* path. You'll get used to it, and you'll start taking it without ever making the conscious decision to do so.

Amidst all this blowing up walls and fighting goblins, there is an important lesson to be learned. While the ultimate goal is getting through the dungeon, every action you take to get there is a smaller goal to be met. Every barrier you trample through is an opportunity to prove to yourself that you are capable of overcoming obstacles. In isolation, they seem small and insignificant. Yet, as they pile up, they contribute toward a sense of self-efficacy. Not to be confused with self-esteem and self-worth, self-efficacy is the belief that we have in our ability to overcome challenges and accomplish our goals (Akhtar, Ghayas, & Adil, 2013). It is the belief that we are *capable*. It has been linked to optimism, subjective well-being, and it is one of the most critical components of achieving meaningful, enduring change (Karademas, 2006).

In the end, change comes from having clear, simple, yet challenging goals in mind, deciding on the path that will get you there, and repeatedly making the choice to move in that direction. Yes, there may be one step forward and two steps back. Yes, your previous experiences and predispositions may impact your journey, for better or for worse. Yet it is always within our power is to take a pause, press reset, and choose a different way. In the end, you will discover not only that you have changed, but how very capable you are of change.

When It's More Than Just a Game: The Impact of In-Game Decisions

While the previous metaphor may seem detached from our everyday experiences, the implications of our in-game decisions reach far beyond the game itself. Our emotions and behaviors change based on what we do during gameplay. This provides us with an incredible advantage to leverage our in-game time to see real-world changes.

A 2014 experiment by Grizzard and colleagues studied the relationship between virtual-world immoral behavior and its real-world effects. Participants were placed on one of two teams: either a guilt-inducing condition (playing the game as a terrorist) or a control condition (playing the game as a UN soldier). Those who played as terrorists reported experiencing greater guilt after the fact and increased feelings of violating their moral values. This study, among others, suggests that social behaviors people enact in the gaming realm can elicit emotional responses much like real-world behavior does. We play a game, and it makes us feel a certain way. Those feelings can and do result in behaviors, in- and out-of the gaming space.

For example, playing relaxing or cooperative video games has been shown to cause increases in pro-social behavior and decreases in anti-social behavior (Dolgov, Graves, Nearents, Schwark, & Volkman, 2014; Whitaker & Bushman, 2012). Playing video games with specifically pro-social narratives (like *Lemmings* and *City Crisis*) has been found to encourage pro-social behavior, from something small (like helping someone pick up pencils) to something much more impactful (like intervening in a harassment situation; Greitemeyer & Oswald, 2010).

These behavior changes can be explained in part by the thoughts we have during gameplay (Greitemeyer & Oswald, 2010). As we play video games, our thoughts are consumed with the tasks at hand: *I should do this, I'm trying to do that, I need to do this.* When we dedicate ourselves to repeated tasks, we are immersing our brain in those thoughts. And as we learned earlier in this chapter, that dedicated brain-space leads to lasting changes in the ways we think and behave.

These findings have huge implications in video games with moral decision making, like *Skyrim* or *Fable*. In these games, we are often presented with key decision points: help or harm. Engage or avoid. Support or ignore. Sometimes, they're face-valid and quite straightforward. (Think about one of the first quests presented to you in *Fable I:* you catch a married man flirting with another woman. Do you accept his bribe and stay quiet, or do you tell his wife?) Some tasks, however, are not so apparent.

> You complete a dungeon raid with some match-made players. A rare piece of armor drops at the end. What you own is better, but you *could* sell it in the forums. You notice another player in your raid could use the armor. What do you do? Do you take it, or leave it?

> You're coming up on a boss fight. You've read the playthrough, you've leveled up, and on paper, you are absolutely ready. But…you're still scared. You think about every way this could go wrong, everything you could lose if you die in this fight. What do you do? Fight or Flee?

> Your friends have picked up a new game. They are having a blast with it, but you are struggling. It seems like fun, but the controls are unfamiliar to you. You're not used to this type of game. You're not improving as quickly as you want. What do you do? Call it quits, or persevere?

In video games, we experience an endless stream of these decision points. They happen constantly—in our interactions with the game narrative, with NPCs, with other players, and even in the task of gaming itself. In open-world games, the possibilities of those decision points are innumerable. Taken in consideration with everything else in this chapter, it's hard to deny: It really is more than just a game.

So let's look back to our scenarios from the start of the chapter: our friend with anxiety, our friend with trauma, and our friend who struggles with emotions. How might they use this framework to work on these concerns?

> *I'm venturing into this new area of the map. There* could *be high level monsters there to kill me…*
>
> *…I'm scared, and that's okay. But rather than think about all the ways that would wreck me, let me instead practice thinking of what the evidence suggests, and make a decision based on that.*
>
> *I'm meeting all these new people in my guild, and I'm not sure how I feel about it…*
>
> *…Why don't I take some time to think about what positive friendships look like and how to set healthy boundaries, so I can feel comfortable getting to know them better.*
>
> *Whenever I play games with my friends, they tell me I'm toxic and they don't want to play with me anymore. (I don't really get it – I'm just giving them feedback, right?)…*
>
> *…But maybe I can ask them to explain why my comments hurt them, and what I can do better.*

…It's definitely not as easy as pressing a button, but it's not so hard as you might think. And video games can be a way to get us there.

References

Akhtar, S., Ghayas, S., & Adil, A. (2013). Self-efficacy and optimism as predictors of organizational commitment among bank employees. *International Journal of Research Studies in Psychology, 2*(2), 33–42.

Bioshock [Video game]. (2007). Boston: Take-Two Interactive, 2K Games.

Burgoon, J. K., Stern, L. A., & Dillman, L. (1995). *Interpersonal adaptation: Dyadic interaction patterns.* New York: Cambridge University Press.

City Crisis [Video game]. (2001). New York: Take-Two Interactive.

Damian, R. I., Spengler, M., Sutu, A., & Roberts, B. W. (2018). Sixteen going on sixty-six: A longitudinal study of personality stability and change across 50 years. *Journal of Personality and Social Psychology, 117*(3), 674–695.

Dolgov, I., Graves, W. J., Nearents, M. R., Schwark, J. D., & Volkman, C. B. (2014). Effects of cooperative gaming and avatar customization on subsequent spontaneous helping behavior. *Computers in Human Behavior, 33,* 49–55.

Entertainment Software Association. (2018). *2018 essential facts about the computer and video game industry.* Retrieved from https://www.theesa.com/wp-content/uploads/2019/03/ESA_EssentialFacts_2018.pdf.

Entertainment Software Association. (2019). *2019 essential facts about the computer and video game industry.* Retrieved from https://www.theesa.com/wp-content/uploads/2019/05/ESA_Essential_facts_2019_final.pdf.

Fable [Video game]. (2004). Redmond: Microsoft Game Studios.

Greitemeyer, T., & Osswald, S. (2010). Effects of prosocial video games on prosocial behavior. *Journal of Personality and Social Psychology, 98*(2), 211–221.

Grizzard, M., Tamborini, R., Lewis, R. J., Wang, L., & Prabhu, S. (2014). Being bad in a video game can make us morally sensitive. *Cyberpsychology, Behavior, and Social Networking, 17*(8), 499–504.

Harwood, T. M., Beutler, L. E., & Groth-Marnat, G. (2011). *Integrative assessment of adult personality.* New York: Guilford Press.

Hughes, C. M., Griffin, B. J., & Worthington, E. L., Jr. (2017). A measure of social behavior in team-based, multiplayer online games: The Sociality in Multiplayer Online Games (SMOG) scale. *Computers in Human Behavior, 69,* 386–395.

Jackson, William A. (2001). A short guide to humoral medicine. *Trends in Pharmacological Sciences, 22*(9), 487–489.

Karademas, E. C. (2006). Self-efficacy, social support and well-being: The mediating role of optimism. *Personality and Individual Differences, 40*(6), 1281–1290.

Lemmings [Video game]. (1991). Liverpool: Psygnosis, SunSoft.

Locke, E. A., & Latham, G. P. (1990). *A theory of goal setting & task performance.* Englewood Cliffs, NJ: Prentice-Hall.

MacLeod, A. K., Coates, E., & Hetherton, J. (2008). Increasing well-being through teaching goal-setting and planning skills: Results of a brief intervention. *Journal of Happiness Studies, 9*(2), 185–196.

Mount, M. K., Barrick, M. R., Scullen, S. M., & Rounds, J. (2005). Higher-order dimensions of the big five personality traits and the big six vocational interest types. *Personnel Psychology, 58*(2), 447–478.

Roberts, B. W., Jackson, J. J., Fayard, J. V., Edmonds, G., & Meints, J. (2009). Conscientiousness. In M. R. Leary & R. H. Hoyle (Eds.), *Handbook of individual differences in social behavior* (pp. 369–381). New York, NY: Guilford Press.

Tang, W. Y., & Fox, J. (2016). Men's harassment behavior in online video games: Personality traits and game factors. *Aggressive Behavior, 42*(6), 513–521.

The Elder Scrolls V: Skyrim [Video game]. (2011). Rockville: Bethesda Softworks.

Tupes, E. C., & Christal, R. E. (1961). Recurrent personality factors based on trait ratings. USAF Personnel Training Research, 57–125. Lackland Airforce Case, TX; Aeronautical Systems Divisions, Personnel Library.

Vygotsky, L. S. (2004). Imagination and creativity in childhood. *Journal of Russian & East European Psychology, 42*(1), 7–97.

Whitaker, J. L., & Bushman, B. J. (2012). "Remain calm. Be kind." Effects of relaxing video games on aggressive and prosocial behavior. *Social Psychological and Personality Science, 3*(1), 88–92.

World of Warcraft [Video game]. (2004). Irvine: Activision Blizzard Entertainment.

Yee, N., Ducheneaut, N., Nelson, L., & Likarish, P. (2011, May). Introverted elves & conscientious gnomes: The expression of personality in world of warcraft. In *Proceedings of the SIGCHI Conference on Human Factors in Computing Systems* (pp. 753–762). ACM.

Zillig, L. M. P., Hemenover, S. H., & Dienstbier, R. A. (2002). What do we assess when we assess a Big 5 trait? A content analysis of the affective, behavioral, and cognitive processes represented in Big 5 personality inventories. *Personality and Social Psychology Bulletin, 28*(6), 847–858.

CHAPTER 3

Explore the Map

Shane Tilton

Abstract This chapter explores the importance of navigating the terrain of social interactions, being open to new experiences, and avoiding the traps of going through the linear motions of the well-worn pathways of life. The rewards for choosing to explore the boundaries of the territory will also be discussed as well as how to minimize interpersonal risk by being able to recognize potential the dangers are and how to react to them. Examples from various games, along with Face-Work and Affect Theory, will be creating an understanding that being open to new experiences means viewing emotion as the pallet that influences a person's views of the world and creates a roadmap of how to be a more open person.

Keywords Face-Work · Affect Theory · Emotional development · Social interactionism · Interpersonal communication

S. Tilton (✉)
Ohio Northern University, Ada, OH, USA
e-mail: S-Tilton@onu.edu

R. Kowert (ed.), *Video Games and Well-being*,
Palgrave Studies in Cyberpsychology,
https://doi.org/10.1007/978-3-030-32770-5_3

Those lucky individuals who owned a Nintendo Entertainment System (NES) and had a subscription to Nintendo Power at the end of 1989 were rewarded with both the game "Dragon Warrior I" and a guide to help play "Dragon Warrior I" (Oxford, 2018). This rare moment of generosity by Nintendo promoted not only the role-playing genre on the NES, but embedded in the minds of video game players the value of a game guide and, most importantly, the need for maps in complex gaming environments. The gaming ecosystem was evolving beyond the linear nature of side-scrollers to interactive play that demanded that the players be aware of their situation and how to navigate through the various digital worlds. A single folded sheet of glossy paper could be the difference between saving the kingdom or becoming lost in the World of Alefgard (the Kingdom that acts as the primary location for "Dragon Warrior I").

The map was more than a way to orient a location within the field of play. Alefgrad's map provided the knowledge of which enemies a player would face at a given site within the game, the coordinates of the critical treasures needed to beat the game, and the waypoints to hit during the various quests within the game. This safety net allows players to be open in their gameplay as they can find the right pathway back to the comfort of the known. This simple tool allowed the player to make the right connections between the gaming terrain and the end goals. They could see how to finish the game and earn their final reward.

A map of this quality is like Linus' blanket from Peanuts. It provides comfort to the nervous soul. Each decision a player makes has been tried, examined, and completed by experts. They can explain what actions the player need to take to get the best armor in the game or how to beat the final boss of the game. Maps like the one found in the "Dragon Warrior I" guide would be helpful to have in the real world, but such a simple tool doesn't exist. Interactions in the realworld are much harder to navigate. Interactions, unlike the Kingdom of Alefgrad, that are not finite in nature. These newer experiences that a person faces on a daily basis do not fit neatly onto a carefully designed map to show how to transverse these various social and cultural decisions making it easy to fall into the traps of going through the linear motions of the well-worn pathways of life and rarely making changes.

It is known, therefore it is safe.

Players also know that the biggest rewards are often outside the realm of the known. There are few opportunities to gain treasure or wealth in the various towns and villages of Alefgrad. Valuable materials on a map are there for people brave enough to explore beyond the safety of the town walls and go into the unknown of the wild. People will only find true rewards by facing their fears and visit the wilderness surrounding the civilized area of the kingdom. Rewards come to those in the game that have access to a good map of the area and the ability to read the dangers along the way and know how to negotiate those potential harms. The same can be true in the real world. A useful guide that can help navigate this balance is one that incorporates social awareness with the ability to perform an emotional self-diagnostic. This type of manual or map uses emotions as the legend to translate how feelings influence our world views. This type of map can help developing a new pathway toward openness to experiences and others.

The purpose of this chapter is to create a version of these beautiful infographics that have long been available for video games for our daily lives. One that can help us to navigate one of life's biggest challenges: to create a balance between the risk of social failures and the reward of social acceptance. Put another way, to balance the emotional well-being of ourselves and others.

This balancing act is a typical battle that a person goes through on a daily basis. Buddhists describe this battle to maintain a sense of emotional well-being as the "second arrow" (De Silva, 1990). The metaphor goes along the lines of a person is walking through the woods and is shot by an arrow. The archer lines up a second shot. The first arrow can be thought of as the social failure a person experiences. The incoming second arrow is the emotional response to that failure. By avoiding that second arrow, a person avoids the emotional trauma of reliving the social failure. Only by avoiding those second arrows can a person enjoy the rewards associated with being accepted by others in society. A person can avoid these traumas by having a guide that helps to show them the way.

On the following pages, two theories are outlined which will create the foundations for the creation of such a map. One that provides landmarks to aim toward (building off the discussion from Chapter 2 in this volume) and the knowledge of how to avoid the barriers along the way. A personal map allows an individual to move forward with the knowledge that they can feel comfortable with the terrain and know how to avoid the barriers that can prevent the successful completion of their goals. In a game, the map can lead to cool armor and treasure. In the real world, a mental model can lead to a life where the person is more open to try new experiences.

Building Your Map via Affect Theory

Creating a personal "map" (much like the maps in video games) can help to develop one's openness to new experiences by providing a base from which to develop a sense of self-worth and level of self-awareness. Put another way, it creates a starting point to grow from.

Affect theory (Tomkins, 1991) is one social theory that can help explain this development. This theory states that there are multiple tiers of affects or emotions that a person can experience. A person can view their feelings almost like a pallet with the ability to craft an understanding of how their experiences will influence their view of the world. Each emotion that a person experiences will tend to shade their view of the world. All of this shading creates an emotion-based mental map of how a person should interact with others. A person that understands the mental map metaphor will be more apt to take a step back and control their more basic emotions for the purpose of understanding their relationship to the overall environment in which they are living (Damasio, 2004) and attempt to take control of more decisions during the course of their everyday existence (Bortolan, 2011). This awareness of feelings or affects is vital as it is part of a person's ability to perform the socially acceptable biological and neurological reactions to a given stimulus (Tomkins, 1991). One example that shows a socially acceptable biological and neurological reaction is laughing at a joke. One example that shows a non-socially acceptable biological and neurological reaction is laughing at a funeral. The former situation is a time and place that laughter would be allowed and normal. The latter situation would be considered taboo to laugh. A person dealing with the spectrum of various emotions and affects often needs a good model for processing this information.

To illustrate how to affect theory works in our daily lives, let's turn to an example from the video game *The Legend of Zelda: Breath of the Wild* (Nintendo) and the relationship between the main character (Link) and his ability to navigate a foreign terrain.

Affect Theory and Breath of the Wild

Link wakes up at a location he doesn't recognize after being in a 100-year coma. His memories are gone, and he has no sense of why he is there (even though the player would know if they are familiar with the series or have played previous games in the series). He must depend on the Sheikah Slate to act as his map of this strange environment. The Sheikah Slate also serves as a sensor to find the temples that improve the health (via Spirit Orbs) or gear of Link. Spicy peppers and mushrooms can be found via the Slate when he has found one in the past and taken its picture, thus giving him the ingredient he needs for the meals and potions of protections. This tool also can act as a form of security by alerting Link when Guardians are nearby, one of the biggest threats in the game. All of these elements that the Slate tracks in the virtuality of the game can relate to real-world interactions.

Humans tend to use stimuli to make sense of the world much like the Slate's ability to ping elements on the map helps the player make sense of the gaming environment. Emotions tend to color and filter reactions to those stimuli. These reactions can impact a person's ability to understand their world.[1]

In Breath of the Wild, knowing where raw meat, spicy peppers, Hyrule Bass, and a cooking fire can help a player create a Spicy Meat and Seafood Fry dish, which will get Link a warm doublet from the Old Man and protection from the cold. In the real world, knowing how to make or buy a meal can reduce the chances of being angry due to hunger pains. A player or person is practicing the basics of self-care by attempting to take care of their basic needs.

Feeling Bubbles

The idea of using recipes to take care of the needs of the individual directly relates to one of the core components that makes up the affect theory. People go through "feeling bubbles" (i.e., emotional connections to specific times; Wetherell, 2014) throughout the course of a given year that is related to the cultural and social moments (e.g., New Year's Eve celebrations and the grief experienced during September 11). People who know the cultural and social terrain during a given feeling bubble and are able to seek and find the resources to practice the basics of self-care related during a given feeling bubble (e.g., if one is an alcoholic, a person might want to know which parties and social gatherings will be alcohol-free during New Year's Eve). A player practices similar aspects of self-care in *Breath of the Wild*.

[1] For example, being "hangry," or being angry due to hunger, is a classic example of emotions coloring a person's view of the world.

One example is when the Blood Moon appears. It is the time where all of the enemies that Link has defeated in the past 28 days of game time are reincarnated, forcing Link to battle these demons again. Players can sense the tension and fear this bubble causes as the game designer invokes a sense of being afraid through effective music that leaves a player feeling on edge and animation reminding the player the horrors that are coming back from the dead. Knowing where a player is on the map can prevent the player from being surprised by the enemies that are now rising from the ground. Using a journal or other tracking device can help Link find the best time to go to an inn and avoid the horror that is the Blood Moon.

Players that use these practices in the game can apply them to the real world to deal with the feeling bubbles and the awareness of the affect a person feels during these feeling bubbles. Self-awareness is the key to best deal with a time of stress and uncertainty (Callan, Terry, & Schweitzer, 2007). Even without a perfect map or guide, a person can attempt to be prepared and aware of their emotional state.

Affect Theory and Minecraft

A more apt representation and simulation of how to map out the social and cultural terrain using affect theory might be from *Minecraft* (Mojang). *Minecraft* is a more open-world experience than *Breath of the Wild* as the player is responsible for maintaining and creating most of the elements that appear within the world of *Minecraft*. The *Minecraft* terrain, and therefore the map, can be changed at a moment's notice based on the destructive or creative nature of the person playing the game. This control of the map by the player speaks to the level of agency a person has in the two games (Frasca, 2010). Players are given a quasi-open world with a finite number of quests and actions they can take to complete the final goal designed by the creators of *Breath of the Wild* to beat Calamity Ganon/Dark Beast Ganon and save Hyrule. The players of *Minecraft* are not limited by any narrative structure created by the game designers as it seems there's not an overarching plot or narrative flow, but rather shared social experience that occurs among those that play *Minecraft* (Schifter & Cipollone, 2013). It is this distinction that can help a person create an emotion-based mental map of their world.

The first step needed for development of these type of maps is understanding the tools needed to create the map. In *Minecraft*, a player needs the right crafting recipe to produce a map, which is eight papers and one compass placed on the crafting table. The real-world counterpart to this could be talking to professionals, reading academic work, or building a support group of people that are going through similar experiences.

The second step is exploring the terrain to filling in the blanks of the terrain. A player uses the game control to fill in the blanks on the map in *Minecraft* to see all of the geographical components of the terrain. A person in the real world can use journaling or use other documenting tools to see how their emotions change based on stimuli experience by the person every day.

The last step in this process is to analyze the terrain. Creating a map room can provide this perceptive in the game. Talking to a professional about the experiences from the journal can help in the real world.

Both maps are colored by the landscape and the person's interpretation of what the landscape means (e.g., "Will I be attacked by Creepers if I go to those blocks in the middle of the map?" or "Will seeing this person make me feel too anxious or scared?"). Both maps require a keen level of insight to understand how to navigate with the least amount of harm and possibly the most sense of fulfillment possible given the nature of the terrain.

Face-Work

Erving Goffman (1985) developed the theory of Face-work as a means of understanding how a person maintains a consistent series of social interactions within a community. These actions are called "maintaining one's face." A classic example of maintaining face in society would be waving to every passing car as a person is driving to maintain the impression that a person is a friendly member of a given community. Maintaining one's face allows that person to be more confident with themselves and more self-assured that they can exist successfully in a given community. One of the critical aspects of Face-work theory that relates to video game mapping is the concept of how a person performs dignity (i.e., the ability of an individual to present their physical and emotional state in social interactions while maintaining their face; Brown & Levinson, 1978) in the real world. These rituals can be a simple as offering food to one member of a community and performing polite small talk (Bucar, 2012) to an individual showing solidarity with others in that individual's community (Bargiela-Chiappini, 2003). Dignity is vital as the act of dignity provides a vantage point that an individual can use to view the rest of the social terrain.

A map is useless if a person can not see where they are in relationship to the rest of the terrain. Any type of emotional mental map or model is equally meaningless if the person cannot maintain some sense of who they are. Dignity provides a person that grounding.

The ground can be shaky in the real world as any emotional mental model must deal with the dynamic social environment that a person is likely to face on a daily basis. A person must recognize that they will be dealing with people whose moods and behaviors will change based on their own "feeling bubbles" (Wetherell, 2014), past experiences (Schein, 2003), or any number of social, psychological or cultural stimuli that can influence the behaviors of the individual on a daily basis. Any model must be prepared for these dramatic changes. Creating such a mental model is illustrated through visiting new planets in *No Man's Sky* (Hello Games).

Face-Work and No Man's Sky

No Man's Sky (Hello Games) provides an example of applying a map to a dynamic landscape. The game engine uses a procedural generation model for creating all of the in-game elements, which means that no two players will have the same map playing the game. There are possibly millions of different variations of monsters, planets, and spaceships that a player will experience over the course of the game (Alexandra, 2016). This layer of complexity also means that it is impossible for there to be a guide that can help a player find new terrain or determine the threats and rewards they will face throughout the course of playing the game. This kind of map is the most similar to the one we experience in our daily lives.

Just like in the real world, a player in this game must study the movements and rituals of the different creatures they will face during the course of the game to determine if those creatures are a threat, harmless, or helpful. The reading of the actions of this computer-generated being begins to provide a foundation for a player to judge the non-verbal mode of communication that other people have in the real world and determine how those people will react to a person's actions and intents.

Advantageously, *No Man's Sky* is also training its players in performing Face-work is when a player goes through the Atlas Path. Atlas Path is one of the side quests that a person can choose to follow in order to understand the mythology of the game. Beyond the functional component of the Atlas Path adding more directions to go on the Galactic Map, the Atlas Path trains a player to understand the influence of societal institution as part of social interactions. Monoliths are placed throughout the map, and the players must learn how to interact and exist with the locations to advance their view and knowledge of the world. Each monolith within the game reveals another part of the underlying story of the game when the player finds those points and interacts with them. A person that is able to find and map these points in the universe is able to understand their place within the game. This mapping is not unlike how a person maps social and societal actions that a person might take on a daily basis.

Mental Mapping the World

Mapping the vital parts of life, much like mapping out the environment of a video game world, involves having a clear understanding of the terrain that is being mapped out. In *Breath of the Wild*, a crafted map that a player can find online can be used to show the player all of the shrines in Hyrule and the pathways that they can use to reach those places. Away from the gaming environment, a person that reaches out to professionals can use those professional's guidance to create mental models and map out the important "feeling bubbles" of their lives. Discussing these "feeling bubbles" with psychologists, psychiatrists, social workers, and other mental health professionals can help lay out the mental landscape of an individual.

Another core component of map creation is that the map must have a clear legend that explains what all of the symbols and signs mean within the cartographic artifact. A good player's map in *Minecraft* will use symbols to show where to find resources. A great player's map will allow the player to tell a story within the landscape. Real-world models must denote what the different "feeling bubbles" mean to a person based on past experiences, memories associated with those "feeling bubbles," and professional guidance on how to deal with those events. The legend represents not only the geography of the land and the barriers that make up the geography, but also the resources that the geography has to offer.

When the world becomes too much, we must seek out the resources that can help.

The final component of map creation in both video games and mental health is the need to ground the map in the reality of the world. Some of the best maps present the aesthetics of the game onto the paper (e.g., the paper map gave with the "Dragon Warrior I" was an excellent example of maintaining the branding of the game with their font selection and maintaining the gaming experience with the graphic layout of the map).

Other great diagrams make the pathways clear between the points of civilization and show the boundaries of the wild world where only the brave dare to travel.

This realism of the world presented on an easily accessible resource can make all the difference in surviving the chaos of the realm. Professionals that can show the critical area to discover in the field and the explorers of the domain can point out the changes that are needed on the map to reflect the reality of the world. Professionals in this example are played by psychologists, psychiatrists, social workers, and other mental health professionals, while the explorers are either those that have experience stress and other issues in society and share those experiences with psychological professionals or those that journal their issues and reflect on those experiences later. This type of mapping of the real world is necessary as a means of not trying to sugarcoat the struggles we all experience or minimizing the pain we can all experience from time-to-time.

The world can be made a better place with one more safety blanket in your hand.

References

Alexandra, H. (2016, October 18). *A look at how no man's sky's procedural generation works*. Retrieved January 17, 2019, from https://kotaku.com/a-look-at-how-no-mans-skys-procedural-generation-works-1787928446.

Bargiela-Chiappini, F. (2003). Face and politeness: New (insights) for old (concepts)☆. *Journal of Pragmatics, 35*(10–11), 1453–1469.

Bortolan, A. (2011). *A phenomenological discussion of Antonio Damasio's theory of emotions*. Retrieved January 13, 2019, from http://www.fupress.net/index.php/pam/article/viewFile/19652/18193.

Brown, P., & Levinson, S. (1978). Universals in language usage: Politeness phenomena. In E. N. Goody (Ed.), *Questions and politeness: Strategies in social interaction* (1st ed., pp. 56–311). Cambridge: Cambridge University Press.

Bucar, E. (2012). Saving face: Navigating land mines with ritual politeness in Iran. *History of Religions, 52*(1), 31–48. https://doi.org/10.1086/665962.

Callan, V. J., Terry, D. J., & Schweitzer, R. (2007, September 25). *Coping resources, coping strategies and adjustment to organizational change: Direct or buffering effects?* Retrieved January 13, 2019, from https://www.tandfonline.com/doi/abs/10.1080/02678379408256543.

Damasio, A. R. (2004). *Looking for Spinoza: Joy, sorrow, and the feeling brain*. London, UK: Vintage Books.

De Silva, P. (1990). Buddhist psychology: A review of theory and practice. *Current Psychology, 9*(3), 236–254.

Frasca, G. (2010, August 9). *Rethinking agency and immersion: Video games as a means of consciousness-raising*. Retrieved May 31, 2019, from https://www.tandfonline.com/doi/abs/10.1076/digc.12.3.167.3225.

Goffman, E. (1985). On Face-work: An analysis of ritual elements in social interaction. In B. G. Blount (Ed.), *Language, culture, and society: A book of readings* (2nd ed., pp. 222–247). Long Grove, IL: Waveland Press.

Oxford, D. (2018, March 29). *Howard Phillips speaks on Dragon Quest's initial performance and Nintendo Power giveaway*. Retrieved January 13, 2019, from https://web.archive.org/web/20190103193927/www.oldschoolgamermagazine.com/howard-phillips-speaks-on-dragon-quests-initial-performance-and-nintendo-power-giveaway/.

Schein, E. H. (2003). On dialogue, culture, and organizational learning. *Reflections: The SoL Journal, 4*(4), 27–38.

Schifter, C., & Cipollone, M. (2013, March 25). *Minecraft as a teaching tool: One case study*. Retrieved May 31, 2019, from https://www.learntechlib.org/p/48540/.

Tomkins, S. S. (1991). *Affect, imagery, consciousness, Vol. 3. The negative affects: Anger and fear*. New York, NY: Springer.

Wetherell, M. (2014, September 5). *Tears, bubbles and disappointment—New approaches for the analysis of affective-discursive practices: A commentary on "researching the psychosocial"*. Retrieved January 13, 2019, from https://www.tandfonline.com/doi/abs/10.1080/14780887.2014.958399.

CHAPTER 4

Oh Me, Oh My! Identity Development Through Video Games

Sarah Sawyer

Abstract This chapter discusses how players interact with, influence, experience, and embody their avatars through gameplay and how this type of exploration can influence development, identity, and social navigation. Particular focus is placed on identity development within video game play, how particular facets of identity (e.g. gender, personality) are malleable in this context, and the styles of exploration via types of games. Considerations of personalized characters, as well as their application to real-world behavior and approach to life, are discussed.

Keywords Avatar · Narrative · Identity

When I opened up my brand-new copy of *Middle Earth: Shadow of Mordor* (Monolith Productions, 2014), I was ecstatic when there was actually a female avatar to play. Of course—as a self-identified lady—I chose this

S. Sawyer (✉)
Take This, Seattle, WA, USA

R. Kowert (ed.), *Video Games and Well-being*,
Palgrave Studies in Cyberpsychology,
https://doi.org/10.1007/978-3-030-32770-5_4

character and embarked on the exciting adventure through the *Lord of the Rings* environment I knew and loved.[1] When I got to the first cut scene, the male protagonist (and other option for an avatar) appeared on screen. As he gallantly defended his family as they were attacked by Uruk, I questioned my choice—did I really choose the female character? Did I button mash and mess it up? Do I need to restart? Nope… even though I could play the game as a female, the cut scenes revolved around *his* story. I found myself feeling irritated about this situation. I questioned if I should continue playing the game. Little did I know, later on, I'd meet my own avatar as a non-player character and have to actually complete missions with her (a bit short-sighted in design, no?). I realized I felt cheated as a player of this game—though I felt more empowered and represented as a female through my avatar, this was not fully fleshed out in the game itself. It was only during non-story-related content that I could engage as the lady brawler. It harkened back to feelings I've had for most of my life as a female human in the world. I reflected about this as I engaged in non-game life things, realizing that I was living out my passion for female empowerment and representation when I reacted to the game. To the experience I had while playing my character… to the disenfranchisement I felt when my character was not whole. My moral stance was getting poked by the structure of its design.

Now don't get me wrong. This is not a chapter about reviewing games, nor is it about equality. It's about the reactions we have and the things we learn about ourselves as we play video games through the avatars we control within them. No, avatars aren't just blue bio-experimental mishmashes of human and alien species—they're the characters we choose to represent us in video games (unless you're playing an *Avatar* game, of course). When selecting characters, video games offer a wide variety of options. Not every game is equal in this regard. Regardless, however, there's an opportunity to self-explore in nearly any avatar. After all, as research shows, the choice to spend time playing video games has a large influence on our wellbeing—so let's make the most of it (Padilla-Walker, Nelson, Carroll, & Jensen, 2010).

This chapter will discuss identity exploration, the specific ways that players use games to explore themselves, and how gameplay can impact the way

[1] I still love it… just felt the game was a bit off the mark for LoTR universe quality.

they conduct themselves in real life. It will explore the way players personalize their characters, engage in play, and how they connect with game narrative as a way of understanding its impact on their lives.

Identity Formation and Exploration

Erik Erickson, the psychologist who coined the phrase *identity crisis*, created a model of how identity development theoretically works (Kroger, 2017). He believed that to understand one's identity is to be able to feel as if one has a purpose, and to have relative consistency in sense of self over time and setting.[2] His theory was that an identity is established through nature, nurture, and social experiences; though maturity does theoretically achieve some stability, he considered that identity development continues over time (Erickson, 1968).

Erickson's (1968) general structure is that people mature through eight stages of development over their lifetime.[3] During each stage, two conflicting ideas must be resolved before an individual can move forward moving on to the next stage of development. The inability to do so leads to feelings of inadequacy and may prohibit an individual from becoming a confident, functional member of society.

The fifth of Erick's stages is of most importance in this chapter. Stage five is called *identity vs. role confusion,* pertaining to the cyclical nature of how people explore their past and current identities, what feels genuine and authentic to them, and considering critically how challenges to their self-concept ought to be integrated… or not (Erickson, 1968). Erickson's theory considered that stage five of development occurs over adolescence and that at identity remains flexible—at least to a degree (Erickson, 1968). Identity research flourished since Erickson's work, and the data supports his theory into modern conceptualization (Kroger, 2017).

Waterman and Archer (1990) considered how the construct of identity is vital to understanding how it develops—particularly through its form, function, and process. *Form* is how a descriptive or role identity is considered, like what religious beliefs or job that someone has. The *function* of an identity provides people with several conveniences, including a sense of

[2] Basically the same theoretical idea as personality.

[3] The eight stages are trust vs mistrust, autonomy vs. shame/doubt, initiative vs. guilt, identity vs. inferiority, identity vs. role confusion, intimacy vs. isolation, generativity vs. stagnation, and integrity vs. despair.

direction, purpose, potential, continuity, and interpersonal presentation of self. *Process* is how identity develops over the lifespan (Waterman & Archer, 1990). When combining the works of Erickson, Waterman, and Archer, we can see how video games provide a unique opportunity to challenge their self-concept without immediately changing their real-life form or function. But wait, Dr. Sawyer, you say—how does any of this apply to video games anyways?

Well, let's back it up to adolescence again. Konijn and Bijvank (2009) consider that role models are crucial to the developmental process. In the virtual space, there are a multitude of characters to consider for this presence in adolescents' lives (Konijn & Bijvank, 2009). Their argument relies on the concept of *social learning theory*—the idea that observing others, and subsequently modeling their attitudes and behaviors, will teach people how to behave based on the reaction they get to the modeling (Bandura, 1977). In the context of identity construction, Konijn and Bijvank (2009) apply four factors that underlie this process through video game play: wishful identification, mastering challenges, immersion and presence, and perceived realism. *Wishful identification* replicates the social learning theory, where players idealize the role models they see in-game. *Mastering challenges* is pretty much what it sounds like… players are faced, inevitably, with a challenge to overcome to progress through the game. The player's role model engages in this challenge, offering players a view of a successful other who overcomes. *Immersion* is the sense of being in the game, mentally losing your physical context—*presence* is the temporary sense of being the avatar you're playing. Consider presence like a next level to empathy, that you're walking in that person's shoes. Finally, *perceived realism* is how real the game environment appears to the player (Konijn & Bijvank, 2009). Integrating along, this means that though this occurs during adolescence, this process of self-exploration and comparison to characters continues with age.

Role models aren't the only way this type of embodiment can impact player identity, as "the virtual self is a somewhat idealized actual self" (Bessiére, Seay, & Kiesler, 2007, p. 531). *Self-discrepancy theory* purports that our wellbeing is significantly tied to the distance that we feel exists between our actual selves and our ideal selves (Higgins, 1987). In application of self-discrepancy theory, Bessiére et al. (2007) discovered that players engage in imagined actualization of the ideal self through play as their avatars, thus reducing the discrepancy between their real and idealized selves. Trepte and Reinecke (2010) argue that this idealized version of ourselves may not look exactly like we do—sometimes, avatars may look and be entirely different from ourselves.

Players are very likely to engage in this automatic "merge" with their character's identity while playing, as their self-perception shifts into the avatar to engage with the game (Klimmt, Hefner, & Vorderer, 2009). To tie things together neatly, this is that presence we were discussing earlier. Included in this merge are self-perceptions, such as attitudes and goals, and social perceptions, such as interpersonal respect, successfulness, and attractiveness (Klimmt et al., 2009). The level of interactivity that video games provide (in lieu of watching something like television) adds to and shapes the player's concept of self by fulfilling the character's role through play (Klimmt et al., 2010).

Look at Me Now—Character Customization

Not all video games allow for the customization of avatars, but instead offer a character (another name for avatar) whose appearance is pre-determined. This was true for the vast majority of video games at their advent (in the late 1970s), and I doubt many of us felt a compelling attachment to the little bar we used to compete in *Pong*. As time went on, game developers began providing a few avatars to pick from, such as in games like *Mario Kart* (Ninendo, 1992) or *Minecraft* (Mojan, 2011). In these games, players are given a choice of avatars who looked different but largely performed the same in-game.

Klimmt and colleagues (2009) relate the categorization of games into three degrees of freedom in virtual roleplaying. The least amount of freedom involves pre-determined avatars like in *Pong*, where the player is connected to the avatar based on empathy and parasocial connection. This is the way we naturally attach emotionally to characters we witness in media (such as my strong hatred for Jeoffrey's character from *Game of Thrones*).

The moderate level of freedom games can offer allow players to have some influence on the story or avatar, though many elements are predetermined for the player (Klimmt et al., 2009). While players are limited in their identity exploration with pre-determined avatar choices, there is another vital element in games relating to player experience: the story. There is a variation on how much control players have over the story, when to move forward in it, and how it unfolds. Sometimes, players can completely control how their adventure progresses—while in other games, they're forced to follow along without any autonomous choices at all. Over time, video games have expanded beyond the simplistic and minimal freedom given to players.

The discrepancy between pre-created and customizable characters—and their stories—is a major influence on identifying as a character compared to identifying with a character (Shaw, 2014). Pre-set stories and characters give players the opportunity to explore their emotional reactions to the character's choices, the actions players are forced to take, and to experience the story most similar to a book. Take, for example, Link from *The Legend of Zelda* (Nintendo) series. He is a "neutral" avatar of sorts. We never hear him speak in any game, only hearing the occasional grunt of when he attacks or lands hard on his feet. Though we cannot change the storyline of the games, we will occasionally get the opportunity to pick how to respond to NPC questions or prompts. In *Breath of the Wild* (Nintendo, 2018), the open-world format game of the series, we get to pick when to go where and what to do. We still have to fight Ganon in the end—but at least it's on our schedule, right?

As games become more elaborate, the realm of character customizability becomes ripe with creative opportunity. The final degree of freedom contains this category of games where players have control of the look and feel of their character, the skills they develop, and the way they play through the game (Klimmt et al., 2009). This affords players two primary categories in which they personalize their gameplay experience—appearance and skill. A game that exemplifies these is *The Elder Scrolls V: Skyrim* (Bethesda, 2019). The process of customizing your character is one that reflects real-world identity exploration, where we decide what to wear and what color to make our hair. We engage in both social learning theory and self-discrepancy, finding an idealized way of representing ourselves. Or, as Trepte and Reinecke (2010) suggest, we try something different entirely.

As an example, let's explore the character creation in *The Elder Scrolls V: Skyrim* as a mirror to our own personal identity exploration. When I completed this activity myself, I created my character to be strong in negotiation and social charm—probably because I have a tendency to put a foot in my mouth![4]

[4] Not actually, that'd be VERY disgusting. Also—a footnote is very meta, no?

In-Game Identity Exploration as a Mirror to Who We Are

In *The Elder Scrolls V: Skyrim* (Bethesda, 2019), you start the game from a first-person perspective; your character's gender, race, and voice are unknown. A non-player character (NPC) asks how to address you, and you enter the customization menu (that is elaborate to say the least). You're offered several races to pick from, each with a particular naturally enhanced skillset. Let's say you pick your race as a Khajiit (a wildcat-humanoid avatar). They are excellent at sneaking, pickpocketing, and lockpicking (Bethesda, 2019). Depending on which race you select, there will be a shift in the way you're treated in different regions of the land—for example, Khajiit is subject to discrimination due to their beasty looks and stereotypes about their ability to thieve (Sukkau, 2012). Once you've got your race selected, you can modify the body of your character in a multitude of ways. From cheek bones to tattoos, height to nose. You select the shades and patterns on your avatar's skin (or fur, in your case,) gender,[5] hair, and name. Let's say you chose a lady you name Scooper for your beloved avatar; hey, maybe you're silly. You do you, friend. End cutscene, return to a dragon attack, and Scooper gets the heck out of there just in time to begin her journey.

In-Game Appearance as Identity Expression

Now, let's pick at some of this for a minute before we continue with Scooper's adventure. *Skyrim* is one of many games where players can alter their avatar's appearance in a great variety of ways. It's important to consider how we can explore ourselves through the way our character looks to us and to others (given we're playing multiplayer or online formats). It is one of the fundamental elements of the way, in the real world, we communicate information about ourselves (Villani et al., 2016). Perhaps weight is of concern, or height; maybe you're self-conscious about how you dress and wish you could really wear that Orcish armor (it is, after all, always in style). In the media we consume, in the messages we hear from family and friends, and in the daily onslaught of advertisements, we are spoon fed a lot of information about how we're *supposed* to be. How we're supposed to express ourselves. There's a lot of rules and guidelines imposed upon us that limit us, drag on us like hiking with a backpack that's a bit too full and there's many miles yet to go. The freedom of video games is that we can

[5] Unfortunately, it seems that female and male are currently the only options.

escape these restrictions—lose the backpack from our weary shoulders and get hiking with new energy.

Let's lean on the private, almost vulnerable, sense that video games provide. You can try on a different appearance than you have in real life—it's just you that is aware of this situation; if it's not only you, then everyone else is doing it too (can't shame the neighbor you run into next to the hemorrhoid cream at the store, know what I mean?). Perhaps, if you're a petite and short-statured person, try playing a tall and muscular Orc. If you're quick-witted, try playing an avatar with lower intelligence that has to make up for it with physical ability or dexterity. If you feel defeated in your life at work or school, play a character that looks vicious or intimidating, powerful or threatening—one that will command a room simply with their presence. Bessiére, Seay, and Kiesler (2007) studied this very concept—finding that regardless of the rules and constraints that games put upon us, the anonymity games provide allows players to shed their real-life environment (and self) in favor of a more ideal virtual experience.

To really poke at that vulnerability, I want to tread into the waters of gender. Layers, remember? Gender expression in games hasn't always had the best reputation (see the introduction to this chapter), but there are opportunities to do something different with this too. Maybe it's unsafe to try dressing or expressing a gender different from your natal sex. Maybe you don't feel comfortable taking that step and are curious about your own gender identity or the expression of it. Games can help you to test the theoretical boundaries of gender expression through the characters you can play. In Shaw's (2014) text, participants in her study on identity and gameplay shared that their characters helped them feel validated in their gender experience. Maybe try some *Lara Croft: Tomb Raider* and see what a strong woman feels like at play—not because she's cute, or sexy, or whatever other superficial factors are attributed to the video game icon—but because she perseveres and fights for her life and does not succumb to the negative messages she receives about her ability as a woman.

No, I don't think games will fix the world—but maybe they can be one small thing to bring a moment of joy to your life. Of course, there is also the fact that some games perpetuate the system that oppresses—encourages Whiteness, masculinity, and all the real-world privileges that come with the "majority" statuses. If you find yourself playing a game that does this, I hope that those who reap the benefits of privileged status can consider and recognize this within the game—and that those who suffer oppression can do what they need to take care of themselves when they play. Step away if you have to. I hope that more and more folks in the community can continue advocating for diverse and rich storylines, characters, and abilities so we can heal and grow from games as an activity rather than hurt.

For those with physical limitations, such as a disability or injury, games could provide an opportunity for feelings independence, freedom, and empowerment. Trepte and Reinecke (2010) found that players preferred to use avatars that were dissimilar to themselves when they experienced less satisfaction with their day to day lives. They also found that personality similarity was more important to players to physical similarity. Games could also lean on the oppression bit about how most games provide representation to able-bodied folks… Not to sound like a broken record, but take care of yourself. Let the game be a tool for you rather than a source of pain or another echoing reminder of where you're at in life. Lean on games with characters that help you feel positive, empowered, and energized. Validated. For able-bodied folks, remember—let's continue advocating for diverse and inclusive game design so we can all play characters that empower us—whatever format that may be. We're crossing a bit into the physical application category, so perhaps we ought to transition to the skills category of customization.

I Got Skills

The skills your character has and can develop may very well be your method of expression rather than anything vain at all. Perhaps you're the type of player who chooses the character not for what they look like, but for what they can do. Maybe this even influences the types of games you choose to play in the first place. Reflect for a moment on why you play games (or are interested in playing them). Do you want to feel like you're accomplishing things since you feel stuck or have little control over things in real life? Do you play for a break? Your purpose can play a large part of how you approach character development in a game. Madigan (2016) revealed in his book how our avatars can positively influence our behaviors based on their in-game behaviors—from exercise to confidence and task completion. This is emphasized when the avatar looks even a little bit like us. Perhaps you want to cooperate with characters, befriend them—quell feelings of loneliness or social isolation. Klimmt et al. (2009) found that this is helpful due to the interactivity that games provide. Maybe you like to watch the world burn and want to just punch everything and everyone since in real life you really can't do that.[6] Maybe you want the game to be like a book—a story to experience, a way to relax and enjoy. Perhaps it's a way to be socially relevant or present with folks you can't typically see or talk to without them.

Morals also steer your choices in games. Grizzard et al. (2014) studied the way we emotionally react when playing with immoral choices (willful terrorism). They discovered that when players performed immoral acts, their moral sensitivity increased (Grizzard et al., 2014). In the newly-released first chapter of the game *Deltarune*, you go through the trouble of personalizing your character just for the game to tell you it doesn't matter what name you choose, or what your character likes to eat, or even its favorite color… the implication is that the player's behaviors are what matter—not what the character looks like on the screen. The choices players make are what make or break the game. In its predecessor, *Undertale*, your entire storyline and NPC dialogue changes based on your play style. Do you defeat or spare your foe? Do you befriend or ignore pleas for help? The story (and even ending) evolves with you as you play.

Let's pick back up with Scooper to consider skill choices further. In Scooper's story where we left off, she's free to the world of Tamriel—Skyrim's land where players are set to adventure. You will choose along Scooper's journey who she will affiliate with, what sector of government she'll fight for (if at all), and how she'll treat others. We know Scooper has a natural inclination to be sneaky, is good at getting into locked places, and grabbing goodies from the pockets of unknowing NPCs. The beauty of a game like *Skyrim* is that you don't need to enhance any of the natural skills that Scooper has; you can enhance anything you like. Characters in *Skyrim* have the ability to develop several hierarchies of skill. Players can master enhancements including level of armor protection, amount of weight you can carry, persuasion, archery, magic (both restorative and destructive), and more. As you level up, all of it becomes easier and better.

Perhaps you choose for Scooper to be skilled in alteration—a way in the game to increase your awareness of physical environment. This could apply to your life in the real world by giving you perspective on how you observe what's around you. How aware are you of what's ahead? Behind? Were you checking your cell phone just now? Are there people talking around you, or are you alone? Was that a knock on the door? How distracted are you? Aren't you supposed to be reading?

[6] I mean, you could, but there'd be consequences.

Scooper needs to be able to survive since there are bears and mammoths and dragons (oh my!) around in Tamriel. Perhaps you choose to enhance her one-handed combat skills so she can still perform her alteration magic as you navigate the world. This is a catch-22 if you know anything about managing combat; fighting with a one-handed weapon means you'll have to fight for longer to fatally wound your foe, but you'll waste less energy. You'll struggle with flying enemies, or those far away from you, but you'll be quick and more versatile with moves. These are the little things that players have to consider—what is your interpersonal style? How does it translate into your gameplay? Do you approach interpersonal conflict with a gentle touch? Hang back like an archer? Go in swinging like an Orc with a sledgehammer? Perhaps struggle when you go in too aggressively or too late? As you play, consider how this translates for you. Does your play style reflect your interpersonal approach? Worth and Book (2015) found that personality influences the approach we naturally take when playing games.

We've got Scooper set to be aware of her environment, good at sneaking about, decent at hand-to-hand combat, and let's imagine you choose one more skillset to enhance along your journey as you level up in the game. Perhaps you pick speech as a focus so Scooper can talk her way through any pinch. Luck and sneaking only go for so long, right? Speech and persuasive skillsets often challenge players to work with the nuance of social interaction. This can be a great place to try out different approaches. Are you forward? Would you say the same things your avatar said in the game, but in real-life context? Would you feel confident, judged, or something else entirely? Could you be as suave as Scooper clearly will be by the end of our playthrough? Consider how your character interacts with NPCs or how you choose to interact with others in a multiplayer context. Though often considered a more diplomatic gaming approach, there's a lot to learn during the social pieces of gaming.

Multiplayer Mode

In the context of multiplayer gaming, avatars provide varying levels of anonymity for players to socially engage with one another. Through that safety, I encourage you to consider how you can challenge yourself to grow in ways you feel unwilling in real life. Perhaps you are socially anxious, unsure of how to start conversations or come off as nonchalant to the person you admire. Maybe you wish to be more confident (or at least appear it) to your boss or someone who intimidates you. Perhaps you feel like you're too reactive and wish for more social tact. Playing multiplayer games offer you the unique opportunity to walk "into" or "out of" the spaces shared with real humans represented by their avatars at any time. It's like the social reset button—you can walk away and start over any time. Suler (2004) calls this the *disinhibition effect*, where people are less likely to feel restrained by the social norms we have in face-to-face contexts. Instead, people report feeling freer, act out more often, and say things they normally wouldn't say (Suler, 2004). Feel like you're failing? Challenge yourself by sticking around. Too uncomfortable? C'est la vie! Take a break if your emotions get in the way. Feel like bonus points? Ask if they think you're awkward… just be sure to remember not to feed the trolls. This is not a guaranteed positive and safe space since we add in the free will of others who are also playing with you.

Similar to the earlier discussion of self-exploration in the individual format, ask yourself—why play multiplayer games? Some choose to play because they enjoy the experience of competition and potentially winning. Others play to cooperate and accomplish missions with others. It is an opportunity to show people a character you completely customize, personalize, and that represents what you want them to see of you. In verbal interactions, some people use voice modification or a robotic voice to personify their perfect avatar yet further. Others will use their true voice or simply not chat at all. What does this mean about yourself? How do you wish to represent, if at all, your avatar in real life and yourself in the game?

You, the Authentic Scooper, and Playing Your Best Self

Video games take, arguably, less bravery than the real world to explore a new identity. A quote from Tynes' (2007) chapter about real-world impact of play puts it best:

> We live in the real world, and our lives are full of real problems and joys. When works of interactive storytelling can teach us how to solve those problems and discover those joys, while entertaining us just as novels, movies, and music do, these works become worthy of real cultural critique and join the great conversation of human thought. Such engagist work can utilize and expand our knowledge, immerse us in real ideas and cultures, and provide tools to explore behaviors and interpret events. Art, knowledge, performance, and imagination intersect therein and bestow profound gifts. (p. 227)

My challenge to you, in reading this book and this chapter, is to play as a character radically different from yourself. Try playing as an avatar that is so different that it feels foreign to you. Follow a story that makes you uncomfortable.[7] Play a game that challenges your understanding of yourself and makes you stop to ask—how would I react to this? How does this impact me? What should I do? What would I *really* do? Play a character as close to you in real life as possible. Try things in-between. The goal is to discover what feels *authentic* to you. What feels *inauthentic* to you. Try to find what feels strange, not you at all, not something you like, or something you love (and might not even have expected it). Challenge your own story, your origin, and how you interpret your life.

Try developing skills that you wish to have in the real world through practice in the game. Play characters that take risks you wish you could, or who have personality qualities you wish you could embody. Thrive through your character. The avatars we play in games can become pieces of ourselves—facets of the self, of our personalities, of our thought processes. We can welcome those pieces of our characters and their stories into the way we navigate the real world. They can help us to know ourselves, what it feels like to be authentically us, and how we can be in the world as a result.

References

Bandura, A. (1977). Self-efficacy: Toward a unifying theory of behavioral change. *Psychological Review, 84,* 191–215.

Bessiére, K., Seay, A. F., & Kiesler, S. (2007). The ideal elf: Identity exploration in World of Warcraft. *Cyberpsychology & Behavior, 10*(4), 530–535. https://doi.org/10.1089/cpb.2007.9994.

Bethesda. (2019). *Elder Scrolls V: Skyrim.* Retrieved from https://elderscrolls.bethesda.net/en/skyrim.

Erickson, E. H. (1968). *Identity, youth, and crisis.* New York: W. W. Norton.

Grizzard, M., Tamborini, R., Lewis, R. J., Wang, L., & Prabhu, S. (2014). Being bad in a video game can make us morally sensitive. *Cyberpsychology, Behavior, and Social Networking, 17*(8), 499–504.

Higgins, E. T. (1987). Self-discrepancy: A theory relating self and affect. *Psychological Review, 94,* 319–340.

[7] Not *too* uncomfortable… just aim for out of your comfort zone. I trust your judgment. You have, after all, read this far!

Klimmt, C., Hefner, D., & Vorderer, P. (2009). The video game experience as "true" identification: A theory of enjoyable alterations of players' self-perception. *Communications Theory, 19,* 351–373. https://doi.org/10.1111/j.1468-2885.2009.01347.x.

Klimmt, C., Hefner, D., Vorderer, P., Roth, C., & Blake, C. (2010). Identification with video game characters as automatic shift of self-perceptions. *Media Psychology, 13,* 323–338. https://doi.org/10.1080/15213269.2010.524911.

Konijn, E. A., & Bijvank, M. N. (2009). Doors to another me: Identity construction through digital game play. In C. M. Ritterfeld, M. Cody, & P. Vorderer (Eds.), *Serious games: Mechanisms and effects* (pp. 179–196). New York, NY: Routledge.

Kroger, J. (2017). Identity development in adolescence and adulthood. *Oxford Research Encyclopedia,* 1–23. https://doi.org/10.1093/9780190236557.013.54.

Madigan, J. (2016). *Getting gamers: The psychology of video games and their impact on the people who play them.* Lanham, MA: Rowman & Littlefield.

Padilla-Walker, L. M., Nelson, L. J., Carroll, J. S., & Jenson, A. C. (2010). More than just a game: Video game and Internet use during emerging adulthood. *Journal of Youth and Adolescence, 39,* 103–113. https://doi.org/10.1007/s10964-008-9390-8.

Shaw, A. (2014). *Gaming at the edge.* Minneapolis, Minnesota: University of Minnesota Press.

Sukkau, S. (2012). Understanding the "other": Racism in Skyrim. *Venture Beat.* Retrieved from https://www.humblebundle.com/games/indie-playstation-rebundle-2019?hmb_source=navbar&hmb_medium=product_tile&hmb_campaign=tile_index_7.

Suler, J. (2004). The online disinhibition effect. *Cyberpsychology & Behavior, 7*(3), 321–326.

Trepte, S., & Reinecke, L. (2010). Avatar creation and video game enjoyment: Effects of life-satisfaction, game competitiveness, and identification with the avatar. *Journal of Media Psychology, 22*(4), 171–184. https://doi.org/10.1027/1864-1105/a000022.

Tynes, J. (2007). Prismatic play: Games as windows on the real world. In P. Harrigan & N. W. Wardrip-Fruin (Eds.), *Second person: Role-playing and story in games and playable media* (pp. 221–228). Cambridge: The MIT Press.

Villani, D., Gatti, E., Triberti, S., Confalonieri, E., & Riva, G. (2016). Exploration of virtual body-representation in adolescence: The role of age and sex in avatar customization. *SpringerPlus, 5*(740), 1–13. https://doi.org/10.1186/s40064-016-2520-y.

Waterman, A. S., & Archer, S. L. (1990). A life span perspective on identity formation: Developments in form, function, and process. In P. B. Baltes, D. L.

Featherman, & R. M. Lerner (Eds.), *Life-span development and behavior* (Vol. 10, pp. 29–57). Hillsdale, NJ: Lawrence Erlbaum Associates Inc.

Worth, N. C., & Book, A. S. (2015). Dimensions of video game behavior and their relationships with personality. *Computers in Human Behavior, 50,* 132–140.

CHAPTER 5

Forever Questing and "Getting Gud"

Jamie Madigan

Abstract This chapter focuses on how games encourage us to adopt a growth mindset and develop the grit needed to persist and learn from failure. Many games require persistence and growth—in skills, confidence, knowledge, or tactics. These games apply well-worn models for ramping up player achievement and teaching us how to succeed. Furthermore, digital games require us to embrace failure as paths to success instead of dead ends of frustration and demotivation. In life, as with digital games, defaulting to a growth mindset is extremely adaptive because it assumes that the road to achievement is open to anyone who persists, learns from their mistakes, and works hard. This chapter draws on research from motivation, goal setting, grit, deliberate practice, and growth mindset.

Keywords Growth mindset · Motivation · Feedback · Goal setting · Grit · Learning orientation

J. Madigan (✉)
Ballwin, MO, USA
URL: http://www.psychologyofgames.com

R. Kowert (ed.), *Video Games and Well-being*,
Palgrave Studies in Cyberpsychology,
https://doi.org/10.1007/978-3-030-32770-5_5

"Don't wish it were easier, wish you were better."
—Chief from *Animal Crossing* (Nintendo Games)

Being bad at a video game once helped me be a better parent.

A little over two years ago I was driving in the car and chatting with my daughter, who was twelve years old at the time. Opportunities for uninterrupted time alone to talk to her were rare since I usually just sit in my room and play video games whenever I get the chance. So I decided to ask her about the summer swim team we had signed her up for. It was a competitive team with regular practices and competitions almost every week. I asked her if she was looking forward to it.

She said no, which wasn't the answer I was expecting.

"What? Why not?" I asked. "You were into it last summer."

"I dunno," she said, shrugging. "Getting up to practice sucks and the competitions are kinda intense."

Further probing revealed that by "intense" she meant "intimidating" and by "sucks" she means ...well pretty much what you'd think she meant. She's right on both counts, no doubt. The swim meets were demanding competitions pitting her against girls who were often better than her. Many of them were older and had been practicing for longer. Some of them were just more gifted athletes who benefitted from better physiques, longer limbs, and probably gills in a couple of cases. I'm looking at you, Courtney.

But I thought getting excited about competitive swimming would be good for my daughter for all the reasons that caring parents who get to sit comfortably on the sidelines typically do. Physical activity. Being part of a team. Making friends. I really didn't want her to drop out, so I wanted to say something encouraging. I opened my mouth and I almost said exactly the wrong thing at that moment, though. I almost said, "Well, you're really good at it."

But then I remembered: video games.

Specifically, I was thinking of the video game *Dark Souls III* (Bandai Namco, 2016), which I had been diligently working my way through at the time. If you don't know, the *Dark Souls* series is difficult by most standards, but I think most of that reputation is because it brutally punishes you if you don't slow down, proceed with caution, and focus on doing better. While some amount of skill is required—you have to tap buttons and flick thumbsticks at just the right times—it's not sufficient by itself to win. You have to learn how things work, where enemies are hidden, and how to avoid every deadly little trick that the game's designers have created. The game even eschews the whole "reload from a save point" paradigm and makes failure part of the game. When you die, you return to the last checkpoint you rested at and the world resets so that you have to do better on your next attempt. Growth and learning aren't just abstract concepts in these kinds of games; they're practically a mechanic like jumping or inventory management.

My point is that nobody is naturally good at *Dark Souls*. Nobody flies through on their first try if they're truly new to the game. In these and many other types of video games, hardship is an opportunity to learn, an opportunity to persist, and an opportunity to, as they say, "git gud." Video games teach you how to be open to feedback, value improving yourself, and to have what psychologists call a "growth mindset."

Learning to Seek Out and Embrace Performance Feedback

Let's start with how video games encourage us to make use of feedback. Part of the reason why people love video games is that we love getting good feedback about our performance because it helps track our mastery of skills and progress toward goals (Kluger & DeNisi, 1996). We love getting this kind of feedback, but we typically don't get enough of it in our jobs or schools. In the world of work, we get feedback from things like sales figures, annual performance reviews, and maybe some kind of formal measurement of customer satisfaction. At school, we usually have to wait days or weeks to get back grades on assignments or tests. But no matter where you look, the feedback we get is often of dubious origins, mixed in with other things, delayed, or worse. And sometimes we don't get feedback at all.

Not with video games, though. Video games scratch this psychological feedback itch far more effectively. Video games teach us to value immediate, frequent feedback that is focused on outcomes in a way that's usually not threatening. And they frequently make it known how close we are to our goals by providing convenient little progress bars that fill up more the better we do. Video games make us feel a sense of mastery and competence in our best moments, which is something that is central to many models of intrinsic motivation (Ryan & Deci, 2000). These are all things we like and being open to receiving and using feedback to improve other aspects of our lives is a very good attitude to have (Gregory & Levy, 2015).

Psychologists studying how we seek out and react to performance feedback have learned, however, that not everyone reacts to feedback the same way. What's more, some orientations toward feedback are better than others if you want to grow and get better. This concept of "feedback orientation" is usually defined as something along the lines of "an individual's overall receptivity to feedback" (London & Smither, 2002). Some researchers have further broken out this concept and thought of feedback orientation as having five different facets: defensiveness, utility, accountability, social awareness, and feedback self-efficacy (Linderbaum & Levy, 2010).

Defensiveness refers to how much someone likes or dislikes getting feedback. If you wish people would just keep their comments to themselves, you're high on Defensiveness, but if you don't care if people hit you with everything they've got, you're low. Utility refers to a general belief that feedback is important for reaching your goals or creating your desired outcomes. Those who are low on Utility don't see feedback as useful at all. Being high on Accountability means you feel a sense of obligation to act on feedback once you get it (whether you think it's useful or not), while being low on this dimension means you don't feel any particular pressure to act. Those high on Social Awareness tend to use feedback as a tool for understanding what other people think of them while those who are low don't use feedback in this way. Finally, Feedback Self-Efficacy reflects a person's general confidence and comfort level in coping with situations where they are getting feedback.

Video games encourage many of these positive aspects of feedback orientation. As a player, you have to be open to feedback, as it often comes from the mere act of engaging with the game and seeing what happens when you try out various tactics or actions. When playing with other people—be they friends or strangers—we feel some sense of obligation to try and make use of their recommendations if we trust them as a source and see their feedback as given in good faith. And we like to know about our reputation by looking at the kind of feedback and rankings that we get from the game. There is some amount of debate in the psychology literature about the extent to which feedback orientation can be changed through effort, or whether it's a more stable personality trait. But even if it is something that people don't change (or don't want to change), those who spend their free time playing video games have most likely self-selected into a hobby that expects and rewards seeking out and making good use of feedback in order to develop mastery and new skills.

But feedback by itself can only be so motivating. Research has shown that what to really motivate growth and doing well in whatever you're trying your hand at, you should be using that feedback to figure out how to reach the right goal.

Learning to Set the Right Kinds of Goals

One of the most well-researched areas of organizational psychology is goal setting. We know, from a line of research going back to the 1960s, that setting specific, difficult goals increases performance more than having no goals or even having vague intentions of doing well (Locke, Shaw, Saari, & Latham, 1981). If you have people in a factory assembling *Fortnite* (Epic Games, 2017) action figures, you'll get better results if you ask them to make 15 figures in the next hour when they've only done 12 in the previous hour. And this isn't just true of the workplace. It applies to areas like school performance, habit change, athletics, weight management, and many others (Locke & Latham, 2012).

Whatever the context, goal setting work because:

1. Goals focus our attention on what helps us reach the goal and away from things that don't
2. Relative to easy goals, difficult ones require us to increase effort (duh…)
3. Reaching difficult goals requires us to keep that effort up over time
4. Goals encourage us to improve how we do the work instead of relying on what we've done in the past (Locke & Latham, 1990).

Feedback, as described above, is then used to see if there's a gap between where our performance is currently and where it needs to be in order to say we reached the goal. This is called a performance/goal gap. If a gap exists, we ideally work harder, work smarter, or both (Taylor, Fisher, & Ilgen, 1984). The better the feedback and the higher our feedback orientation, the more effectively we can use it to close that gap. You see gamers do this all the time when they figure out how to reach their goal of beating a boss, earning a record time, or winning a match based on the feedback they've accumulated over many play sessions.

But some goals are more effective than others, depending on the situation. Psychologists studying goal setting talk about two broad categories:

performance goals and learning goals. A performance goal is when you set out to achieve a certain outcome. Get such a grade, make so many widgets, run so many miles. They're great because when done right they get results. It's not hard to see how video games make use of performance goals. We see them in progress bars, achievements, and character levels. And quest logs are basically just lists of goals, after all. The open world superhero game *Marvel's Spider-Man* (Insomniac Games, 2018), for example, is rife with performance goals. Everything that you do in that game can be seen as working toward some relatively difficult but very specific performance outcome. Stop all the street crimes. Collect all the backpacks. Take photos of all the landmarks. In other games, even more basic concepts like leveling up a character or finishing a level are treated like goals, with the game painting a very clear picture of where you are, where the goal is, and what you need to do to close that gap. And it's great! It's motivating! Game designers have it figured out!

But it's not the only type of goal that video games have figured out, and it's not the most important type of goal setting that games do in order to encourage a growth mindset. Up to this point I've implied that setting specific, difficult performance goals are more motivating than just saying "Do your best." And this is generally true when the tasks are simple or the person doing them already possesses the skill or expertise needed. But sometimes that isn't the case. Sometimes tasks are new, weird, and unfamiliar. Sometimes they require the person to figure out how to do them. In those cases, learning goals are better than performance goals for not only increasing performance but also for learning new skills.

For example, setting such a goal for a task like stuffing envelopes should lead to better performance. But stuffing envelopes is easy, takes just a few seconds to learn, and can only be done a few ways. Contrast this with an events planner trying to figure out meeting schedules for multiple people across several days when everyone has limited openings on their calendars and different room requirements for their meetings. In cases like this, simply telling people "Figure out how to do your best" works better than giving them a specific, difficult goal. This is because people tend to experiment with different strategies for doing the task, which leads them to optimal approaches and increases their sense of self-efficacy and self-esteem (Seijts & Latham, 2001).

Let's look in more detail at a specific example of how video games can use this kind of learning goal to foster a growth mindset. One of my favorite games in recent years is *Horizon: Zero Dawn* (Sony Interactive Entertainment, 2017). There are so many things to see, shoot, and do in its post-post-apocalyptic open world, and the game is heavily systems driven so that you often have many options and strategies to choose from for any given task. Among the game's virtues is that it has several ways of easing you into things given this complexity. One of these is the hunting grounds, which you can visit in order to complete increasingly difficult challenges.

Every hunting grounds requires you to develop new tactics for killing the robotic animals that inhabit them. Could you just take your bow and plug that Grazer with an arrow? Yes. Sure. That will work. But what if you used your blast sling to startle all the Grazers into a stampede and then shot out the supports from a big pile of logs so that they rolled downhill and killed the whole herd of beasts at once? Yeah! That's way more satisfying, and now you've learned a new trick! And this is the great thing about *Horizon: Zero Dawn*'s hunting grounds: instead of just letting you do what you've always done, they encourage players to improve by developing new strategies that they then carry with them back out into the rest of the game.

The game does this by framing its hunting ground challenges as learning goals instead of performance goals. The NPC dialogue does not tell the player to do anything like "Kill 20 Grazers in two minutes." That's a specific, difficult goal all right, but this is a complex task using weapons and game systems that are still unfamiliar to most players. So the quest givers in the hunting grounds basically say "Kill as many as you can" and the grounds themselves tee up many different possibilities. Which is good! Players should be more motivated to experiment with different strategies and learn the ins and outs of their weapons, abilities, and terrain features. They should, in essence, be motivated to grow and see failure or stagnation as an opportunity to learn something new that will work the next time.

You will see how many other games encourage us to embrace learning goals once you know how to look for it. The *Hitman* video game (Square Enix, 2016) sets up complex locations like a militia compound in Colorado or a fashion show in Paris with hundreds of moving parts and dozens of ways for the player to assassinate the game's deserving targets. Again, shooting them in the back and then running for the exit may work, but the game is specifically designed to reward players for finding new, inventive, and sometimes hilarious ways to bring about their target's demise. Could you drop a chandelier on their head? Make their smartwatch explode? Zap them with an exposed power wire? It all sounds kind of grim (it is an M-rated game about assassinating various villains, after all), but the fun comes in replaying levels and challenging yourself to come up with different ways of reaching your objections. Similarly, *Batman: Arkham City* (Warner Bros. Interactive Entertainment, 2011) gives you a toolbox brimming with different ways to take out The Dark Knight's enemies. You can hit them with a batarang to the face, snatch them while hanging from gargoyles, or pop up from floor grates for a surprise attack, to name just a few. But the boss fight against Mr. Freeze forces you into a learning mindset because he takes several hits to take down and he will only fall for each trick once. If you had always relied on just glide kicks or explosive gel traps, you couldn't beat the boss; you had to find a new approach each time you wanted to attack.

So we can see that video games are excellent at teaching us to adopt learning goals in order to develop new skills and strategies and that they encourage us to seek out and make use of feedback. To the extent that these habits and attitudes are extended to other areas of our lives, we can learn to see challenges and setbacks as opportunities to grow and improve instead of roadblocks that draw boundaries around our talents. We can, in other words, take the lessons of video games and use them to develop a growth mindset.

Games Foster a Growth Mindset

Popularized by Harvard psychologist Carol Dweck in her book *Mindset: The New Psychology of Success*, a mindset in this context refers to attitudes one has about performance, success, and effort (Dweck, 2006). There are two types according to Dweck's research: fixed and growth. Those with a fixed mindset tend to agree with statements like "You are a certain kind of person, and there is not much that can be done to really change that" and "You can do things differently, but the important parts of who you are can't really be changed." Those with growth mindsets, on the other hand, tend to agree with declarations like "No matter what kind of person you are, you can always change substantially" and "You can always change basic things about the kind of person you are."

Those with a fixed mindset tend to believe that they have a stable amount of talents such as athletic ability, intelligence, creativity, or skill at *Mario Kart* (Nintendo, 1992). They're born with that talent. It's their gift from God, genetics, or fate. People who are naturally talented athletes or students, for example, tend to have fixed mindsets about their skills in those areas that set them apart from others. But that's only part of what defines the fixed mindset. Such people tend to further believe that their ability is something to be demonstrated or proven, like dominating on the court or in the leaderboards. Whenever they engage in some task requiring their ability, they feel that they must confirm that they do indeed have the skill by succeeding. And, conversely, fixed mindsets tend to avoid trying something if they think they can't succeed because failure will demonstrate their lack of talent and erode their self-esteem. This attitude can come into play even before success or failure is determined—simply having to work hard on something instead of breezing through it can be seen as a signal that they are lacking. Was running a mile hard for you on your first week of training? Forget running that 5K, you're not cut out for it. Did you have trouble getting an A in Physics 101 as a college freshman? Oooh, better transfer to an easier major because you're not cut out to be an engineer after all. That's the fixed mindset at its worst.

Those with growth mindsets, however, may not necessarily have heaps of raw talent, but they believe that they can improve. They start from the assumption that while some people have more ability in a given area than others, ability in general is something that can improve with effort. They also aren't averse to failing in order to make that improvement happen. People of this type are more likely to see screwing up as a chance to learn how to get better, and they are less embarrassed and frustrated by challenges that are—at the moment—beyond their ability. You only fail when you don't improve over time, and having to try hard on something doesn't mean you're a no-talent loser. It just means you're in the process of getting better at it. When someone with a growth mindset has trouble with a tough class or work assignment, they adapt and try to figure out how to do better instead of trying to find their way into another situation that's not so hard. Such people, Dweck argues, are more likely to be successful, happy, and productive no matter where their reserves of raw talent top out. And organizations that hire employees for potential and are thus characterized by a growth mindset tend to be more innovative, flexible, and risk-taking than those characterized by a fixed mindset (Dweck, 2014).

None of this is to say that those with a fixed mindset are lazy and always stall out early because they quit when things get hard. And it doesn't mean that natural talent is a myth and everyone starts out on a level playing field. Indeed, according to Dweck's research, fixed mindsets may be overrepresented among the elite and super successful, simply by virtue of having more talent or ability. Some people have longer legs, some people have a better head for numbers, some people have faster reaction times. Those professional *DOTA 2* (Valve, 2012) players who won the last International tournament are probably gifted with quick fingers and a frighteningly good ability to switch their attention back and forth between various aspects of a match. But they probably also practiced hard, deliberately sought out challenging games, and maintained a constant belief that they could get better. Because video games are well suited to foster a growth mindset.

Dark Souls III is one example I've already discussed, but any game that gives players a chance to stand up, dust themselves off, and recover from a loss is going to encourage players to develop more of a growth mindset. The first time I went to play a match of the online collectible card game *Hearthstone* (Blizzard Entertainment, 2014), I thought I had the game figured out. Instead, I got wrecked by my opponent for reasons I really didn't understand. It turns out that I had misunderstood the importance and power of some of the game's basic tactics and mechanics, such as using minion cards to soak up damage and empower other cards. Instead of quitting, I thought about what someone with a growth mindset would do. I went back to the tutorial and even looked up a couple of beginner's guides online to figure out what I didn't know and how to get better. I'm not winning any *Hearthstone* tournaments, but I'm better than I was.

And that's the thing about video games: They're designed to give you every opportunity to grow and change. In fact, they require it. Game designers don't stack the decks against players to the extent that they can't win. Generations of players have come to expect that you can ease into something new and challenging, learning how to handle it and progressing toward mastery by increments. If you take the lessons of video games to heart and apply them to other areas of your life, you'll expect to fail, you'll expect to learn from that failure, and you'll expect to get better.

Let's return to the conversation I was describing at the top of this chapter, where I was wanting to convince my daughter to stick with her difficult and frustrating swim team experience. In response to her complaint that swim team was hard and intimidating, my instinct as a parent was to say "But you're good at it!" It would have been true, since she was indeed a strong swimmer. But instead I bit my tongue as I thought about all that research on growth mindsets, learning goals, and positive feedback orientation. And about how my daughter loved to put time into video games like *Team Fortress 2* (Valve, 2007), *Rocket League* (Psyonix, 2015), and her biggest obsession at the time, *Overwatch* (Blizzard Entertainment, 2016). She had started out barely able to work the controls or grasp basic tactics in all of those games, but she had steadily kept at them until she was regularly winning matches and getting MVP accolades. So instead I looked at her and said "Well, you've improved a lot at swimming since you started." And then I told her about that boss at the end of the tutorial in *Dark Souls III*.

As I write this, two and a half years after that conversation, my daughter just finished a great season on her high school swim team. She was, in fact, one of only two freshmen that made the cut for next year's varsity team. She still can't quite outperform most of the older, more practiced swimmers she goes up against, but she'll keep getting up for 5 am practices, listening to her coach's feedback, and getting better. She's a gamer. She understands how these things work.

References

Batman: Arkham City [Video Game]. (2011). Burbank, CA: Warner Bros. Interactive Entertainment.

Dark Souls III [Video Game]. (2016). Tokyo, Japan: Bandai Namco.

DOTA 2 [Video Game]. (2012). Seattle, WA: Valve Corporation.

Dweck, C. S. (2006). *Mindset: The new psychology of success.* New York: Ballantine Books.

Dweck, C. S. (2014). How companies can profit from a growth mindset. *Harvard Business Review*, 28–29.

Fortnite [Video Game]. (2017). Cary, NC: Epic Games.

Gregory, J., & Levy, P. (2015). *Using feedback in organizational consulting.* Washington, DC: American Psychological Association.

Hearthstone [Video Game]. (2014). Irvine, CA: Blizzard Entertainment.

Hitman [Video Game]. (2016). Tokyo, Japan: Square Enix.

Horizon: Zero Dawn [Video Game]. (2017). San Mateo, CA: Sony Interactive Entertainment.

Kluger, A. N., & DeNisi, A. (1996). The effects of feedback interventions on performance: A historical review, a meta-analysis, and a preliminary feedback intervention theory. *Psychological Bulletin, 119*(2), 254–284. https://doi.org/10.1037/0033-2909.119.2.254.

Linderbaum, B. A., & Levy, P. E. (2010). The development and validation of the feedback orientation scale (FOS). *Journal of Management, 36*(6), 1372–1405. https://doi.org/10.1177/0149206310373145.

Locke, E. A., & Latham, G. P. (1990). *A theory of goal setting & task performance.* Englewood Cliffs: Prentice-Hall.

Locke, E. A., & Latham, G. P. (2012). *New developments in goal setting and task performance.* New York, NY: Routledge.

Locke, E. A., Shaw, K. N., Saari, L. M., & Latham, G. P. (1981). Goal setting and task performance: 1969–1980. *Psychological Bulletin, 90*(1), 125–152. https://doi.org/10.1037/0033-2909.90.1.125.

London, M., & Smither, J. W. (2002). Feedback orientation, feedback culture, and the longitudinal performance management process. *Human Resource Management Review, 12*(1), 81–100. https://doi.org/10.1016/S1053-4822(01)00043-2.

Mario Kart [Video Game]. (1992). Kyoto, Japan: Nintendo.

Marvel's Spider-Man [Video Game]. (2018). Tokyo, Japan: Sony Interactive Entertainment.

Overwatch [Video Game]. (2016). Irvine, CA: Blizzard Entertainment.

Rocket League [Video Game]. (2015). San Diego, CA: Psyonix.

Ryan, R. M., & Deci, E. L. (2000). Self-determination theory and the facilitation of intrinsic motivation, social development, and well-being. *American Psychologist, 55,* 68–78.

Seijts, G., & Latham, G. (2001). The effect of distal learning, outcome, and proximal goals on a moderately complex task. *Journal of Organizational Behavior, 22,* 291–307.

Taylor, M. S., Fisher, C. D., & Ilgen, D. R. (1984). Individual's reactions to performance feedback in organizations: A control theory perspective. In K. M. Rowland & G. R. Ferris (Eds.), *Research in personnel and human resources management* (Vol. 2, pp. 81–124). Greenwich, CT: JAI Press.

Team Fortress 2 [Video Game]. (2007). Seattle, WA: Valve Corporation.

CHAPTER 6

Positive Psychology and Gaming: Strength and Resilience +1

Ryan Kelly

Abstract Over the last 20 years, positive psychology has had a remarkable rise within research and clinical practice. More and more, psychologists are shifting from a deficit-focused view of mental health to a strength-based one, proactively focusing on factors like positive emotions, engagement, relationships, meaningfulness, purposefulness, and achievement (i.e., PERMA) instead of just psychopathology. Respectively, this chapter introduces an evolved "dual-factor" model of mental health that includes a positive dimension (i.e., "subjective well-being"), proposes a gaming-based conceptualization of strengths and weakness, and discusses the evidence-based uses of video games within the PERMA model as a way to foster resilience and well-being. Case and practical examples are included.

Keywords PERMA · Dual-factor model of mental health · Positive psychology · Role-playing games · MMORPG

R. Kelly (✉)
Southeast Psych, Charlotte, NC, USA
e-mail: rkelly@southeastpsych.com

R. Kowert (ed.), *Video Games and Well-being*,
Palgrave Studies in Cyberpsychology,
https://doi.org/10.1007/978-3-030-32770-5_6

Humans are problem-solvers. This is the inevitable, paramount prerequisite to becoming the apex organism of our planet's evolutionary hierarchy. Millions of years of developing a superior capacity to identify what's missing, broke, lacking, or dangerous—to imagine hundreds of threatening "what ifs" in a moment to procure a solution or a "better". We are inherently deficit-focused. We want solutions—we *need* them—and so we naturally look for problems to solve. This innate feature is the promethean gift that became "science", and within science, psychology—the study of the brain, the mind, and human behavior. But to what extent does this progress us? How does this paradigm benefit us psychologically?

This chapter will address this issue by proposing an alternative paradigm of mental health (i.e., "positive psychology"), including a more comprehensive assessment tool (i.e., the "dual-factor" model) and an innovative, solution-finding approach using video games to better understand our strengths and improve our well-being, and in particular our resilience (i.e., the capacity to recover from difficulties).

Traditional Model of Mental Health

We have become adept at studying abnormalities of human thought, feelings, and actions. Attention Deficit Hyperactivity Disorder (ADHD), Autism Spectrum Disorder (ASD), Generalized Anxiety Disorder (GAD), Bipolar Disorder, and whatever else can fit on a nametag and be slapped on a person like a "faulty product" sticker. From those abnormalities, we have made assumptions about what is "normal", which is often (inaccurately) viewed as synonymous with "healthy" or "functional". For instance, the traditional model of mental health simply includes the presence or absence of psychopathology (i.e., mental illness) exists on a continuum ranging from well-being on one end and psychopathy on the other.

Does anything stand out to you? Do you already recognize a problem with this model? Beginning with the initial conceptualization and development of the mental health field, psychologists, researchers, and educators have used this deficit-focused approach to identify internal and external variables that negatively affect the psychological well-being of individuals. Similar to the medical model used in the field of physical health, this pathogenic approach is based on a unidimensional continuum theory that postulates positive mental health as the absence of illness or disability (i.e., psychopathology; Keyes, 2005). As a result, the vast majority of mental health research and practices aim to identify and ameliorate psychological symptoms (e.g., negative emotions, psychopathological behaviors, and psychological distress) with little regard for important positive psychological factors (e.g., individual strengths, life satisfaction, and positive emotions). This is done so under the assumption that such amelioration equates to high well-being; that if I am frequently sad, I am clinically depressed; if not, I am clinically happy. To put it simply, "if it ain't broke, don't fix it – it works!" Certainly, it is important to be aware of (and to accommodate) weaknesses and limitations, but is this really the best approach? Is our growth as individuals—as a species—still primarily dependent on nullifying weaknesses? Or has humanity reached a point where we must challenge our deficit-focused source code and pursue something greater—perhaps something more positive and strength-based?

Positive Psychology and Mental Health

This question was first formally addressed in 1948, when the World Health Organization officially recognized the overemphasis on the negative human condition in mental health research, whereby the constitutional concept of mental health was revised to include a positive dimension. At that time, health became newly defined as a state of complete physical, mental, and social well-being and not merely the absence of disease or infirmity (World Health Organization). In the years following this amendment, a new body of literature specific to mental functioning beyond the absence of pathology (see Kelly, Hills, Huebner, & McQuillin, 2012 for a review) emerged to include positive mental health factors such as happiness, gratitude, life satisfaction, and positive attitudes, in addition to pathology (Gurin, Veroff, & Feld, 1960; Veroff, Feld, & Gurin, 1962). Today, research continues to identify and explore concepts within the positive dimensions of mental health, representing an increasingly appreciated theoretical approach known as positive psychology.

To this point, consider a bicycle, laying on the ground with the chain off the gear. We see the problem—the chain is off the gear. We see the solution—put the chain back on the gear. Simple. Now, imagine someone comes by and asks, "what can you do with that bike?" The only response you could provide is "nothing, it's broken". We are hyper-focused on the problem. We do not see that the bike has top-of-the-line suspension to adapt to all terrains. We do not see the lightweight, durable frame that can withstand all weather conditions and structural strain. We do not see the perfectly pressurized, optimized cross-training tires that make the bike

Table 6.1 Relationship between subjective well-being and psychopathology

Psychopathology	*Subjective well-being*	
	High	*Low*
Low	Flourishing	Vulnerable
High	Symptomatic but content	Troubled

exceptional. All we know is that the chain is off the gear and it's "useless", rendering us oblivious to the outstanding potential of that bike. So how might that relate to humans?

Let's go back to that traditional, unidimensional model of mental health, where if one does not have psychopathology (i.e., their "chain" is not off the "gear"), then they are considered to be "fully functioning". Now, let's instead consider an alternative approach—a dual-factor, multidimensional model—where we *also* consider the presence or absence of "subjective well-being" (SWB) (i.e., the other valuable aspects of the bike). Refer to Table 6.1.

Subjective well-being is a modern construct in positive psychology that represents individuals' cognitive assessments of their lives as a whole and is thought to include what allows and motivates individuals to positively engage, experience, and assess their lives in meaningful ways (Diener, Napa Scollon, & Lucas, 2009). Diener (1984) defined SWB in terms of life satisfaction (cognitive appraisal of one's life), adequate positive affect (i.e., frequent positive emotions like happiness, joy, gratitude, etc.), and low levels of negative affect (infrequent negative emotions, such as sadness, anxiety, hopelessness), a dynamic configuration that has recently received a great deal of attention to its importance in mental health assessment.

Research has demonstrated the utility of SWB assessment as a mechanism to understanding the positive aspects of mental health (Kelly et al., 2012). Furthermore, research has consistently shown that youth with higher SWB are more likely to have greater physical and mental health, academic performance, confidence, resilience toward stressful life events, higher self-efficacy and -esteem, and fewer behavioral problems (see Haranin, Huebner, & Suldo, 2007; Huebner, 2004, for review; Lewinsohn, Redner, & Seeley, 1991; Martin & Huebner, 2007; Park, 2004; Suldo & Huebner, 2004). In other words, SWB is a strength-based, powerful and invaluable component of assessment, growth, and intervention. And how might this look within the dual-factor model. What do we find?

Referring back to the deficit model discussed in the introduction, the old assumption would be that there are still only two groups: "flourishing" (low psychopathology, high SWB) and "troubled" (high psychopathology, low SWB)—much like the bike example, either the person is fully functional or they are "broken"—but this is not true. Referring to Table 6.1, we actually find two new, distinct groups: those who are "symptomatic but content" (high psychopathology, high SWB) and those who are "vulnerable" (low psychopathology, low SWB). This has been shown to represent 8 and 20% (respectively) of children and adolescents (Kelly et al., 2012). Even more interesting, studies have found symptomatic but content students demonstrate better resilience, self-esteem, sociability, and engagement than the troubled and (some) vulnerable students, suggesting that SWB can be a more predictive variable of positive outcomes than psychopathology (i.e., the "problem") (Kelly et al., 2012). It reveals that we *must* look at what makes something work well, in addition to what impairs functioning. In a nutshell, this is the essential basis of positive psychology.

Positive psychology is a fairly new, innovative branch in the world of psychology. An often used definition for positive psychology is "the scientific study of what goes right in life (Seligman & Csikszentmihalyi, 2000)". Martin Seligman founded positive psychology to look at the strengths of individuals and communities that assist in helping them thrive. According to Dr. Seligman:

> *There are huge differences between a teenager who is not depressed or anxious and one who bounds out of bed in the morning with twinkling eyes; between an adolescent who says no to drugs and one who says yes to meaningful involvement in family, school, community activities; and between one who costs society little and one who actually benefits* [society]. (Seligman et al., 2005, p. 498)

Instead of only repairing what's bad, positive psychology uniquely builds upon what's good and successful in life (Seligman & Csikszentmihalyi, 2000). Within the field of positive psychology, mental health professionals, and scientists focus on variables like character strengths, well-being, self-confidence, compassion, elevation, and optimism (Ackerman, 2019). It is strength-based! Positive psychologists asks questions like what allows humans to persist? What makes them resilient? What makes trauma survivors experience post-traumatic growth versus post-traumatic stress? What makes relationships work versus fail? As it turns out, these questions are incredibly important to ask. For instance, a Gallup poll found that the successful employees and CEOs stood out among their peers in their awareness and dependence on their own strengths versus an understanding and accommodation of their weaknesses (Flade, Asplund, & Elliot, 2015). In other words, it is often more beneficial to further develop one's strengths more (or at least in addition to) than buffer one's weaknesses.

Conceptualizing Positive Psychology Through Video Games

In this regard, imagine you are beginning a campaign in a video game—let's say a role-playing game (RPG) like *Dark Souls*. For those of you who do not know the wonderful nightmare that is *Dark Souls*, it is a notoriously difficult game where, even after grinding and buffing a character to mortem, level one enemies can still kill you and ensure that you lose ALL of your collected money and "soul", as well as hours of progress. Above and beyond similar massive multiplayer online role-playing games (MMORPGs) like *World of Warcraft* or *Skyrim, Dark Souls* requires cautious planning, teamwork (you can "summon" up to three other players), persistence, and resilience. It. Is. Brutal. To fully grasp the weight of this, you can google "Dark Souls Rage Compilation" and commune our anguish (I have seldom felt more defeated or empowered than when playing this game). That being said, character selection is critical, and players can choose between various classes differing in skill points across attributes, including Vitality (e.g., health points), Attunement (e.g., spell slots), Endurance (e.g., stamina), Strength (e.g., attack power), Dexterity (e.g., action speed), Faith (e.g., miracle magic), Intelligence (e.g., spell magic), and Resistance (e.g., toughness). Let's take a look at the attribute profiles of the starting classes as outlined in Table 6.2.

Among these profiles, I have **bolded** and underlined the significant strengths (+3 points from the average) and **bolded** the significant weaknesses (−3 points from the average). So what do you notice? You may notice that the Deprived, Pyromancer, and Knight have no significant strengths or weaknesses. They have what psychologists call a "commensurate profile", meaning they are "appropriately" developed in each area and will have no exceptionalities on either end. Because of this, they are the easiest characters to play with *at the beginning*. They have enough vitality to take a hit (unlike sorcerers), enough strength to wield an effect melee weapon (unlike thieves), and enough dexterity or intelligence to use low-level spells

Table 6.2 *Dark Souls* classes and attributes

Class (level)	*Vitality*	*Attunement*	*Endurance*	*Strength*	*Dexterity*	*Faith*	*Intelligence*	*Resistance*
Knight (5)	14	10	10	11	11	11	9	10
Wanderer (3)	10	11	10	10	**14**	**8**	11	12
Thief (5)	9	11	9	9	**15**	11	12	10
Bandit (4)	12	**8**	**14**	**14**	9	10	**8**	11
Hunter (4)	11	9	11	12	**14**	9	9	11
Sorcerer (3)	**8**	**15**	**8**	9	11	**8**	**15**	**8**
Pyromancer (1)	10	12	11	12	9	8	10	12
Cleric (2)	11	11	9	12	**8**	**14**	**8**	11
Deprived (6)	11	11	11	11	11	11	11	11
Warrior (4)	11	**8**	12	13	13	9	9	11

and long-range weapons (unlike bandits), but what about as the game progresses? Would we want to ensure a commensurate profile, or would we want to abide by a strength-based, dynamic profile like research suggests? What would be more beneficial? For consideration, let's look at the highest rated *Dark Souls* builds within MugenMonkey Character Builder (a well-respected resource for RPG gamers), including the top 11 out of roughly 1 million proposed builds used by some of the top-rated players (as seen in Table 6.3).

Quite a different table! In the first table of starting classes, only 9% of all the cells represented a significant strength, just 10% represented a significant weakness, and an overwhelming 81% represented a neutral value. However, in the table of the top 11 builds, 31% of the cells represented a significant strength (a 344% increase), 55% represented a significant weakness (a 550% increase), and only 14% represented a neutral score (a 578% decrease)! So it would seem that, much like we've seen in research (e.g., the Gallup poll), primarily investing "points" into strengths versus weaknesses is overwhelmingly more beneficial! As a note, this is true in virtually every competitive and role-playing video game, and is often true in life. However, in the real world, it is not always that simple. In my opinion, there are a variety of mental health conditions that follow a similar trend—a dynamic profile of human strengths and weaknesses—often misunderstood as solely a "disorder". Within a gaming profile of primary attributes like *Dark Souls*, I believe they would roughly look like the attributes in Table 6.4.

Much like in video games, it's going to be easier at the beginning to be (neuro)typical—that is, having a commensurate, balanced ("normal") profile. However, in theory, the "disorder" profiles have a greater capacity to excel in life if they can learn resilience, capitalize on their strengths, and create an environment that downplays or accommodates their weaknesses. Admittedly, this is easier said than done. Perhaps the best way to conceptualize all of this would be through a realistic example. So, let's consider the case of "Cloud", a now incredibly successful 26-year-old client (and gamer) of mine who, like many individuals with ADHD, has a very dynamic profile of strengths and weaknesses.

Cloud is exceptionally creative, and has a great capacity to "hyperfocus" when he's interested in or passionate about something, which allows him to surpass even his greatest peers in work ethic and productivity. This is not uncommon. Individuals with ADHD often score higher in measures of creativity compared to their neurotypical peers (White & Shah, 2011). Furthermore, ADHD is generally misunderstood as an *inability to focus*,

Table 6.3 Top rated builds from MugenMonkey character building

Build	*Vitality*	*Attunement*	*Endurance*	*Strength*	*Dexterity*	*Faith*	*Intelligence*	*Resistance*
Crestfallen Warrior	45	8	40	40	40	9	9	11
Oroboro's Falchion	50	16	40	12	40	30	8	11
OnlyAfro's Bandit	48	12	66	16	10	10	8	11
MarcyM's Bandit	37	8	89	30	9	10	8	11
Weyendyonwiks Warrior	12	8	37	14	14	9	9	99
Chaos Samurai	40	12	40	16	45	8	10	12
SlintEastwoods Pyro	50	16	85	27	10	8	10	12
Oroboro's Cleric	50	14	42	12	40	30	8	11
Artorias v.2	49	10	51	23	23	20	18	11
Rin_Tohsaka	48	12	30	27	40	30	14	11

Table 6.4 Dynamic profile of strengths and weaknesses in *Dark Souls* character building

Diagnoses	*Intelligence*	*Creativity*	*Passion*	*Attention*	*Social skills*	*Executive functioning*	*Emotional regulation*	*Consciousness*
ADHD	11	15	17	6	9	7	8	7
Aspergers	15	10	17	9	5	9	7	10
Anxiety	11	8*	10	11	8	13	6	13
Depression	11	16	16	8	9	8	5	7
Bipolar I	10	17	15	7	9	9	5	8
Neurotypical	10	10	10	10	10	10	10	10

*represents a preference for acting within structure and rules, not necessarily a limitation in creative abilities

when it's actually a limitation in being able to *shift and maintain focus*; meaning, if they are working on something of interest, you cannot stop or distract them! Cloud fits the bill when it comes to this, especially in art and innovative engineering. These strengths make him exceptional.

He is also what we sometimes refer to as "smart but scattered", where he has a genius IQ score (which allowed him to skate by in school despite homework incompletions and procrastination), but also has clinically significant difficulties in inattention, impulsivity, and hyperactivity. Although he could easily get all As in all AP classes, his grades in school were As, Bs, and Cs, as he would literally never finish homework or study. This was because of his notable weakness in executive functioning, referring to his ability to regulate thoughts and attention, to manage his time, plans, and behavior, and to begin, maintain, and complete tasks. His profile might look like Table 6.5.

Because of this, in primary and secondary school, he was often getting in trouble for impulsively blurting or acting out in class, being a class-clown, not paying attention, and not completing his homework. At home, he was often getting in trouble with his parents due to lying about his studies and

Table 6.5 Cloud's dynamic strengths and weaknesses profile

	Intelligence	*Creativity*	*Passion*	*Attention*	*Social skills*	*Executive functioning*	*Emotional regulation*	*Conscientiousness*
Cloud	15	15	17	6	7	5	8	7
Neurotypical	10	10	10	10	10	10	10	10

Table 6.6 Cloud's profile determined by environment

	Attention	*Social skills*	*Executive functioning*	*Emotional regulation*	*Honesty/Obedience*	*Total points*
Cloud	6	7	5	8	6	32
Neurotypical	10	10	10	10	10	50

poor decision-making in regards to house rules, especially with problematic gaming. With peers, they would often sneer, tell him to "stop being so loud", call him weird for being so energetic, and generally reflect to him that he is "annoying, odd, thoughtless, dumb, and immature". Obviously, this was a hard time in his life. He was often poorly appraised by his family, peers, and school according to variables *they* determined to be important based on their culture. Unfortunately for Cloud, those variables put more weight on his weaknesses while virtually neglected his strengths. Without necessarily saying it explicitly, like many kids with ADHD, he was viewed as a disabled product of weaknesses and faults. He was often viewed by others like outlined in Table 6.6.

For a long time, Cloud internalized this deficit-focused reflection of himself. He, too, began to ignore his strengths, as they didn't seem to be important in the world around him, and instead defined himself by his weaknesses. He felt like he was a liar, a bad student, a bad son, a gaming addict, lazy, weird, broken, weak, and worthless. He tried to avoid this pain and the stress of a harsh environment by playing video games, engaging in reckless behavior, and desperately making "hail-mary" attempts to receive acknowledgment and acceptance. This is common for a lot of youth with dynamic profiles of strengths and weaknesses, especially within an education system and a culture that consistently devalues them. Including other aforementioned mental health conditions, such individuals are often seen as seen in Table 6.7.

However, after starting therapy and working hard to set goals, reconceptualize himself and his world, and putting evidence-based tools to work, he excelled! We got him an Individualized Education Plan (IEP) at school to help improve and accommodate his executive functioning, created a firm yet flexible structure at home with a healthy family communication system absent of needless criticisms and power struggles, and got him enrolled in a robotics and engineering group to exercise his outstanding creativity, intelligence, and hyperfocus (an environment in which he received peer acknowledgment and acceptance). We also worked on a way to limit his

Table 6.7 Dynamic profile of strengths and weaknesses across diagnoses

Diagnosis	*Attention*	*Social skills*	*Executive functioning*	*Emotional regulation*	*Total points*
ADHD	6	9	7	8	30
Aspergers	9	5	9	7	30
Anxiety	11	8	13	6	38
Depression	8	9	8	5	30
Bipolar I	7	10	9	4	30
Neurotypical	10	10	10	10	40

use of gaming for the unhealthy purpose of avoiding reality (i.e., avoidant coping), and instead use it proactively as a way to socialize with supportive peers (e.g., Minecraft with friends from our social skills group), exercise (e.g., Zombies, Run! and Pokemon Go), better understand himself (e.g., considering the games he relates to and the choices he makes within them), develop and practice his "ideal self" (e.g., role-playing games), exercise self-regulation (setting SMART goals for anger and screen time management), and incentivize himself (e.g., Habitica, Gamified Task Manager), among other things.

Cut to seven years later, and he is an independent entrepreneur who helps to develop creative and innovative ideas (capitalizing on his strengths), and then sells them to leave the follow-through and executive management to others (minimizing his weaknesses). Although he did need to improve his executive functioning to some degree (something we worked on throughout college), he did not let that distract him from prioritizing, developing, and utilizing his strengths. As a note, he now relies on those who are naturally organized to manage his schedules, emails, and so on, and has fine-tuned his otherwise "annoying" energy and extroversion to generate enthusiasm and inspire investors!

So what can we learn from Cloud's story? How does this tie in what we've previously discussed? Instead of solely focusing on and defining himself by his deficits, he learned resilience, capitalized on his strengths, and found ways to improve *and/or* accommodate his weaknesses. Although he has what some view as a "disorder", he focused on SWB variables as a way to adapt to this, much like the other 8% of his peers within the dual-factor model considered "symptomatic but content". Furthermore, although Cloud did struggle with problematic gaming similar to addiction, his road to success started by learning and practicing a new paradigm—positive psychology—through the conceptual framework of something he loved and understood—video games! And although he needed help developing self-regulation with his gaming use (he went screen-free during the first week of therapy), transitioning back into play video games responsibly and proactively was an essential part of his therapeutic growth! Now, Dr. Kowert and all of the contributors within this book are fully aware of the powerful and therapeutic benefits of gaming, but what is a good way to conceptualize its use through the paradigm of positive psychology?

Applying Positive Psychological Principles to Gaming

Video games have had a common use in the rise of the technological era. Many people have been critical of technological usage for multiple reasons, including social isolation, toxic social environments, skin gambling, loot crates, (mis)reported correlations between gaming and violent or aggressive behavior, and the recent addition of "gaming disorder" as a distinct addiction by the World Health Organization. Parents have been critical of the amount of time their children spend on gaming for fear that it's overwhelming their lives, and there are certainly those gamers whose "problematic gaming use" does encroach upon their domains of life (e.g., school, friends, physical health, etc.). In cases like Cloud's, it'd be insensitive and irresponsible to blame the parents and teachers for harboring concerns. Within research, traditional psychology movements continue to focus on these negative psychological aspects. For example, a common claim and caution derived from research is how video game usage increases aggression (curiously defined as punishing a competitor with a loud sound) in both the short and (theoretically) long term (Anderson & Dill, 2000). Although this can be useful information, ironically, the problem with this unipolar approach is that it only focuses on the problems. It suggests a strong bias against gaming, seemingly operating under the assumption that video games are inherently wrong, when in reality, they're simply tools.

I sometimes equate gaming and gaming technology to nuclear fusion, especially when speaking to parents who are concerned about their child's gaming behaviors. When it comes down to it, both gaming and nuclear fusion are just tools—powerful tools—that can either be harnessed for good (therapy, perpetual energy) or carelessly abused (dependency, hydrogen bombs). The point is, we should not be preoccupied wondering if it's good or bad—that's a moot point—rather, we should be focused on learning ways to harness it! Connecting the world of video games with positive psychology does just that; instead of simply pathologizing a remarkable feat of human innovation, we can show the healthy and constructive utility of gaming, the benefits of which are unique and plentiful. One way to do this is by using Martin Seligman's model for positive psychology, which contains five parts: positive emotion, engagement, relationships, meaning and purpose, and accomplishment. Known as PERMA, researchers can use this model to analyze the benefits of video game usage.

As it relates to positive emotion, players tend to use video games (often violent ones, including *Doom, Dead or Alive, Grand Theft Auto, Mortal Kombat, Resident Evil, Prince of Persia*) in order to better manage their intense emotions of anger, frustration, and stress. In youth studies, players who play a moderate amount of video games (6–10 hours a week) reportedly "let off steam" in a safe and controlled environment, and often do so effectively (Allahverdipour, Bazargan, Farhadinasab, & Moeini, 2010; Kutner & Olson, 2008)! This is sometimes referred to as "sublimation"—a mature coping skill whereby individuals express their unacceptable idealizations by means of appropriate action. In this way, a teen playing *Grand Theft Auto* after a rough day at school would be akin to a businessman punching a punching bag after a contentious day at work.

Furthermore, moderate gameplay has been shown to increase emotional stability and decrease depression and loneliness. This is especially true with immersive games that allow children to play as their ideal selves, where the larger the discrepancy between their actual self and in-game ideal self, the greater the positive emotional effect (Przybylski, Weinstein, Murrayama, Lynch, & Ryan, 2011). Overall, research suggests that even violent video games can have positive emotional benefits when played in moderation (6–10 hours a week) and when done proactively (i.e., the child's aware of his/her emotions and plays specifically to address it). As a note, this does not mean that all violent video games are appropriate or healthy for all ages (for a reference on age-appropriate games, see www.commonsensemedia.org).

Engagement refers to one's emotional involvement or commitment to an interest. Positive engagement is often linked to greater well-being and connectedness with others, and can foster a state of "flow" (i.e., "being in the zone") similar to what we might pursue through mindfulness. The more immersive the game, the more true this becomes, such as when a player begins to personally identify with their in-game character (Shernoff, 2012; Snodgrass, Lacy, Dengah, Fagan, & Most, 2011). As a result, gamers may gain a high sense of empowerment and productivity when their character levels up, such as in MMORPG games like *World of Warcraft*. This has been found to lead to increased self-reports of happiness, stress management, and life satisfaction.

Similarly, we've found that as their characters become stronger and more equipped for new challenges and goals, so can the players (Bardzell, Bardzell, Pace, & Reed, 2008). The truth is, although we must learn to face reality and choose to engage in problem-solving coping, we must also develop healthy avoidance and present-awareness coping skills. These allow us to *temporarily* escape our real-life concerns, especially those that we don't have control over, and instead relax and simply be present. Now, as a noteworthy caveat, the psychological benefits of dissociative or meditative states derived from immersive video games do become problematic as gametime exceeds moderate use. This is a common guideline in video game use, as it is with most things.

Regarding therapy, engagement has also been shown to improve upon the efficacy of existing, evidence-based therapeutic interventions. This is especially true for groups of people who naturally demonstrate high engagement through Special Interest Areas (SIAs), such as those with high-functioning autism or ADHD. For instance, in an experimental study on the effectiveness of social skills groups for "aspies" (those with Asperger's Syndrome), researchers compared a standard social skills group to one that included a social skills computer game. As a note, all of the participants reported having a special interest in computers and video games. The study found that while both groups showed significant gains, only the group that included the video game demonstrated a significant increase in social motivation (Kelly, 2015). By incorporating their natural engagement with computers and video games, the participants also demonstrated an increase in their social engagement.

Relationships have shown to be successful through friends playing video games together, both in person and online (when including online communication). A positive aspect is that gamers often use their gaming community as a safe space to express their appearance, gender, sexuality, or age that they might be too uncomfortable to do in real life. For instance, one study found that two-fifths of participants would discuss sensitive issues with their online gaming friends that they would not discuss with their real-life friends (Cole & Griffiths, 2007). Understandably, this fosters greater intimacy and trust in their gaming peers. Research has found that socializing through the medium of multiplayer games can help both initiate and maintain supportive, meaningful relationships, as well as enhance face-to-face relationships (Valkenburg & Peter, 2011; Williams et al., 2006).

Relationship building is inherent in most video games. For instance, most online multiplayer games (e.g., *World of Warcraft, Fortnite, Words With Friends, Minecraft*, etc.) are explicitly designed to encourage people to engage with one another (sometimes referred to as "stickiness") by providing notifications of other players' activities, recommending friends based upon consistency of gameplay or progress, and creating incentives to work cooperatively and develop teams or "guilds". This social capital has been found to extend beyond the game, as the players genuinely value each other and often regard in-game achievements as simply achievements (Trepte, Reinecke, & Juechens, 2012). In other words, if Jake leads his *League of Legends* team to victory through persistent practice, strategizing, problem-solving and effective communication, he is not just seen as a good gamer—he is viewed as an intelligent, analytical, wise, and persistent leader, even outside of the game. This kind of peer approval can go a long way in terms of self-confidence and -esteem.

The meaning and purpose aspect of why video gaming is so beneficial is primarily that players feel like they are apart of something bigger than themselves. The larger the group of online gamers working together, the more meaning the player gets out it (McGonigal, 2011). This is a general truth when it comes to humans, but specifically with video games, it's because gamers find themselves working with other gamers on difficult challenges. This makes them feel obligated to put in their best effort in order to succeed. We find that this leads to strong online ties, even if they know they are never going to meet up in person with their fellow gamers (Pwn or Die Blog, 2009). Furthermore, by completing challenges, achieving goals, and growing in the game, players may gain a great sense of mastery (especially if they struggle to achieve real-life goals)—a sense of competence and confidence that can generalize outside of the game.

The last part of PERMA is accomplishment, which is often the primary "pull" that keeps gamers playing. In a video game, accomplishing something is regular, achievable, and immediately rewarding. Players receive immediate rewards and recognition when a task is completed, and acknowledge the motivation, hard work and persistence it took to get there (McGonigal, 2011). Players feel highly productive when they achieve their goals, which leads to a positive experience, and enhanced self-worth (Seligman, 2004). Furthermore, video games often provide a structured framework for goal-setting (e.g., first find the prospector, then grind in the woods until your Level 5, then pursue his missing friend) and foster a growth-based mindset (e.g., I'm not proficient enough to fight the Level 30 monsters, but that doesn't mean I can't work hard and progress), which can generalize into real-life goal-setting behaviors. Another sense of accomplishment players report feeling is in building a supportive in-game network; the sense of pride and achievement that comes with helping similar people come together, connect, and have fun.

Concluding Thoughts

It's important to remember that video games are simply tools—wonderful and powerful tools—that despite having a potentially negative impact, also demonstrate an exceptional utility in improving players' well-being. Although as humans we naturally look for problems and are inclined to worry and panic about potential "threats", that does not mean we should ignore the positive elements of what might be used to foster growth and optimal functionality. By design, video games prime us to enter a strength-based mindset (e.g., picking characters based on their strengths, focusing on progress and goals), which naturally allows us to observe positive psychological effects through the framework of PERMA. Within this model, research shows that video games help to increase positive emotions, decrease negative emotions, promote engagement and mindfulness, foster meaningful relationships, instill a sense of meaning and purpose through mastery and belongingness, and provide a blueprint on how to achieve one's goals and, consequently, obtain greater self-confidence, -competence and -esteem.

Through video games, people can enjoy both a sense of social identity and achievement satisfaction that would otherwise be too difficult to achieve, while enhancing their morality through understanding virtual-world rules and effectively strategizing in accordance with them (Tian, 2009; Wang & Liu, 2012). Players can then discuss these strategies with one another, and through competition or cooperation, form a meaningful bond that may extend to a real-life friendship. The relationship between video games and gamers is not a simple human–computer interaction model, but rather a relationship containing discussion, collaboration, and reflection between peers in the form on websites, forums, and other platforms (Williamson & Facer, 2003). There are so many opportunities for gamers to share their love of their games with one another that such benefits continue to be strengthened and influential, even when the game is over and we reenter the real world.

References

Ackerman, C. (2019, July 10). *What is positive psychology & why is it important?* Retrieved from https://positivepsychology.com/what-is-positive-psychology-definition/.

Allahverdipour, H., Bazargan, M., Farhadinasab, A., & Moeini, B. (2010). Correlates of videogames playing among adolescents in an Islamic country. *BMC Public Health, 10*, 286. Retrieved from http://www.biomedcentral.com/1471-2458/10/286.

Anderson, C. A., & Dill, K. E. (2000). Video games and aggressive thoughts, feelings, and behavior in the laboratory and in life. *Journal of Personality and Social Psychology, 78*(4), 772–790.

Bardzell, S., Bardzell, J., Pace, T., & Reed, K. (2008). Blissfully productive: Grouping and cooperation in world of warcraft instance runs. In *Proceedings of the 2008 ACM Conference on Computer Supported Cooperative Work (CSCW '08)* (pp. 357–360). New York, NY: ACM.

Cole, H., & Griffiths, M. (2007). Social interactions in massively multiplayer online role-playing gamers. *Cyberpsychology, Behavior and Social Networking, 10*, 575–583.

Diener, E. (1984). Subjective well-being. *Psychological Bulletin, 95*, 42–575.

Diener, E., Napa Scollon, C., & Lucas, R. E. (2009). The evolving concept of subjective well-being: The multifaceted nature of happiness. In E. Diener (Ed.), *Social Indicators Research Series: Vol. 39. Assessing well-being* (pp. 67–100). Dordrecht: Springer.

Flade, P., Asplund, J., & Elliot, G. (2015). *Employees who use their strengths outperform those who don't.* Retrieved from https://www.gallup.com/workplace/236561/employees-strengths-outperform-don.aspx.

Gurin, G., Veroff, J., & Feld, S. (1960). *Americans view their mental health.* New York: Basic Books.

Haranin, E., Huebner, E. S., & Suldo, S. M. (2007). Predictive and incremental validity of global and domain-based adolescent life satisfaction reports. *Journal of Psychoeducational Assessment, 25*, 127–138.

Huebner, E. S. (2004). Research on assessment of life satisfaction of children and adolescents. *Social Indicators Research, 66*, 3–33.

Kelly, R. M. (2015). *Group social skills interventions for children with Aspergers: The effects of parent-guided social skills software* (Doctoral dissertation). Retrieved from https://scholarcommons.sc.edu/etd/3722.

Kelly, R., Hills, K., Huebner, E. S., & McQuillin, S. (2012). The longitudinal stability and dynamics of group membership in the dual-factor model of mental health: Psychosocial predictors of mental health. *Canadian Journal of School Psychology, 27,* 337–355.

Keyes, C. L. M. (2005). Mental illness and/or mental health? Investigating axioms of the complete state model of health. *Journal of Consulting and Clinical Psychology, 73,* 539–548.

Kutner, L., & Olson, C. K. (2008). *Grand theft childhood: The surprising truth about violent video games and what parents can do.* New York: Simon & Schuster.

Lewinsohn, P. M., Redner, J. E., & Seeley, J. R. (1991). The relationship between life satisfaction and psychosocial variables: New perspectives. In F. Strack, M. Argyle, & N. Schwarz (Eds.), *International series in experimental social psychology, Vol. 21. Subjective well-being: An interdisciplinary perspective* (pp. 141–169). Elmsford, NY: Pergamon Press.

Martin, K. M., & Huebner, E. S. (2007). Peer victimization and prosocial experiences and emotional well-being of middle school students. *Psychology in the Schools, 44,* 199–208.

McGonigal, J. (2011). *Reality is broken: Why games make us better and how they can change the world.* Sydney: Random House.

Park, N. (2004). The role of subjective well-being in positive youth development. *The ANNALS of the American Academy of Political and Social Science, 591*(1), 25–39.

Przybylski, A. K., Weinstein, N., Murrayama, K., Lynch, M. F., & Ryan, R. M. (2011). The ideal self at play: The appeal of video games that let you be all you can be. *Psychological Science, 23,* 69–76.

Pwn or Die Blog. (2009). *12 ways video games actually benefit real life* [Web log post]. Available at http://www./pwnordie.com/blog/posts/15739. Accessed July 21, 2019 [Google Scholar].

Seligman, M. (2004). *Authentic happiness.* New York: Free Press.

Seligman, M. E. P., Berkowitz, M. W., Catalano, R. F., Damon, W., Eccles, J. S., Gillham, J. E., … Peterson, C. (2005). The positive perspective on youth development. In D. L. Evans, E. Foa, R. Gur, H. Hendrin, C. O'Brien, M. E. P. Seligman, & B. T. Walsh (Eds.), *Treating and preventing adolescent mental health disorders: What we know and what we don't know: A research agenda for improving the mental health of our youth* (pp. 497–527). New York, NY: Oxford University Press.

Seligman, M. E. P., & Csikszentmihalyi, M. (2000). Positive psychology: An introduction. *American Psychologist, 55,* 5–14.

Shernoff, D. (2012). Engagement and positive youth development: Creating optimal learning environments. In K. R. Harris (Ed.), *APA educational psychology handbook, Vol. 2: Individual differences and cultural and contextual factors.* Washington, DC: American Psychological Association.

Snodgrass, J., Lacy, M., Dengah, F., Fagan, J., & Most, D. (2011). Magical flight and monstrous stress: Technologies of absorption and mental wellness in Azeroth. *Cultural Medicine and Psychiatry, 35,* 26–62.

Suldo, S. M., & Huebner, E. S. (2004). Does life satisfaction moderate the effects of stressful life events on psychopathological behavior during adolescence? *School Psychology Quarterly, 19,* 93–105.

Tian, W. (2009). The educational potential of online games from a psychological perspective. *Journey of Chongqing University Science and Technology, 2,* 214–215.

Trepte, S., Reinecke, L., & Juechens, K. (2012). The social side of gaming: How playing online computer games creates online and offline social support. *Computers in Human Behavior, 28,* 832–839.

Valkenburg, P. M., & Peter, J. (2011). Online communication among adolescents: An integrated model of its attraction, opportunities, and risks. *Journal of Adolescent Health, 48,* 121–127.

Veroff, J., Feld, S., & Gurin, G. (1962). Dimensions of subjective adjustment. *Journal of Abnormal and Social Psychology, 64,* 192–205.

Wang, D., & Liu, D. H. (2012). Review of correlative research of young people's network game. *Advertising Panorama, 12,* 53–61.

White, H. A., & Shah, P. (2011). Creative style and achievement in adults with attention-deficit/hyperactivity disorder. *Personality and Individual Differences, 5*(50), 673–677.

Williams, D., Ducheneaut, N., Xiong, L., Zhang, Y., Yee, N., & Nickell, E. (2006). From tree house to barracks: The social life of guilds in World of Warcraft. *Games and Culture, 1,* 338–361.

Williamson, B., & Facer, K. (2003). More than just a game: The implications for schools of children's computer games communities. *Education, Communication and Information, 4*(2/3), 253–268.

CHAPTER 7

Gaming the Mind and Minding the Game: Mindfulness and Flow in Video Games

Mark D. Cruea

Abstract Mindfulness has received growing attention in recent years as a method for improving well-being. Closely connected is flow, the state of mind one achieves when completely absorbed in an activity. This chapter explores the connections between mindfulness, flow, and video games. Conclusions show that video games are useful for inducing a flow state, which can lead to mindfulness through relaxation, enhanced concentration, improved mood, reduced stress, and greater empathy. While mindfulness and flow can be achieved through a variety of games, certain video games, such as Playne, have also been developed with the specific goal to improve mindfulness. Given the proliferation of video games for computers, consoles, and mobile devices, video games serve as readily-available tools for teaching mindfulness and improving overall well-being.

Keywords Mindfulness · Flow · Video games · Well-being

M. D. Cruea (✉)
Ohio Northern University, Ada, OH, USA
e-mail: m-cruea@onu.edu

R. Kowert (ed.), *Video Games and Well-being*,
Palgrave Studies in Cyberpsychology,
https://doi.org/10.1007/978-3-030-32770-5_7

Over the last three decades, the word mindfulness has become increasingly prevalent in public discourse. However, it is certainly not a new concept as the term was first used in relation to early Buddhist practices during King Asoka's reign in India circa 270–230 BCE. The practice of mindfulness gained popularity in the West, and the United States specifically, in the late 1970s when Jon Kabat-Zinn introduced Mindfulness-Based Stress Reduction (MBSR) to patients at the University of Massachusetts Medical Center as a way of reducing daily stress (Husgafvel, 2016). Since then, there has been a growing literature on the many benefits of mindfulness training, such as reduced stress, depression, anxiety, and negative thinking, as well as improved mood and increased compassion (Bergland, 2015; Brown & Ryan, 2003; Mayo Clinic Health Systems, 2015). Mindfulness is also often discussed in relation to its ability to impart flow, which is the state of mind one achieves when completely absorbed in an activity (Csikszentmihalyi, 1975; Jackson, 2016). Flow comes with its own range of benefits, including an elevated sense of well-being in organizational settings, police officers' jobs, runners and ultrarunners, and music performance (Drosman, 2015; Ilies et al., 2017; Juncaj, 2017; Martinez & Scott, 2016; Sedlár, 2014).

Over the last few years, research has noted how mindfulness, flow, and well-being[1] are specifically tied to video games (Weber, Huskey, & Craighead, 2017). Given the often-frantic activity involved with playing video games, it might seem counterintuitive to associate video games with mindfulness. However, video games are particularly adept at inducing a state of flow, making them well-suited tools for mindfulness training (both intentionally and unintentionally).

What Is Mindfulness?

Mindfulness is "paying attention in a particular way: on purpose, in the present moment, non-judgmentally" (Kabat-Zinn, 1994, p. 4). It is about focusing on the present moment (Nhat Hanh, 2017). Practicing mindfulness has also been found to have a range of psychological benefits, including improved attention, mood, optimism, self-esteem, and ability to cope with stress, as well as reduced fatigue and anxiety (Frazer & Stathas, 2015; Heckenberg, Hale, Kent, & Wright, 2019; Hoffman, 2010; Kabat-Zinn, 1994, 2002, 2017, 2018; White, 2014). While mindfulness has grown in

[1] For the purposes of this chapter, well-being is defined as the "optimal psychological functioning and experience" (Ryan & Deci, 2001, p. 142).

popularity, modern life in Western cultures largely fosters the opposite: our attention being split between several things at the same time (Pickert, 2014). For example, at work our attention may be split between a report we need to complete and the barrage of emails showing up in our inbox. At home, our attention might be divided between trying to answer a child's question and listening to the nightly news. Right now, your attention might be split between reading this paragraph and the incoming notifications on your phone. When attention is split in this way, it is impossible to be mindful of any one particular experience or moment. However, when fostered and used as a tool, mindfulness can train us to be in the moment, even as these kinds of "split-attention" experiences unfold.

Video Games, Flow, and Mindfulness

Given the fast-paced nature of many video games, it is reasonable to assume that mindfulness is the exact opposite of the experience that is being cultivated from playing them. However, video games are extraordinarily adept at inducing a state of flow (Bowman, 2008; Bowman, Kowert, & Ferguson, 2015; Sherry, 2004), which can be a bridge to mindful thinking and practice. A "flow experience" refers to a situation of complete absorption or engagement in an activity (Csikszentmihalyi, 1990). As further described by Csikszentmihalyi (1990), when in a flow state, "people are so involved in an activity that nothing else seems to matter; the experience itself is so enjoyable that people will do it even at great cost, for the sheer sake of doing it" (p. 4). It is important to note that a flow experience is not the same as intrinsic motivation, which is when someone is motivated to complete a task because it is naturally satisfying rather than for an external reward (e.g., I play video games because I find them enjoyable versus I play video games because I am being paid by someone to do so).

Early on, Csikszentmihalyi applied his theory to games by identifying how a state of flow can be achieved while playing chess, poker, or tennis. Video games, however, seem to be exceptionally well-suited to encourage flow because, by their nature, they meet the four preconditions outlined by Csikszentmihalyi (1993) to induce a flow state.

Provide Concrete Goals and Rules

All games have some type of goal whether that be completing a level, defeating an enemy, collecting loot, or simply exploring an environment.

In *Assassin's Creed Odyssey* (*ACO*; Ubisoft), the playable character has the ability to level up after enough points through in-game interaction and achievements. These ability points act as another type of goal since the points can then be redeemed for additional character skills. As well, when a quest in *ACO* is accepted, clear directions are provided to help the player complete the quest and once the quest is complete, the result is shown on screen through text as well as accompanying music that celebrates the achievement.

Actions that Adjust to the Players' Capabilities

This is where video games begin to stand out from traditional games in their ability to induce flow states as video games allow for an optimal balancing of system challenge and skill (Bowman, 2008; Sherry, 2004). For example, *ACO* allows the user to choose from easy, normal, hard, and nightmare difficulty settings, and players can manually readjust the level of difficulty at any point during the game. The game also includes level scaling, which enables the user to set the enemy's difficulty in comparison to the player's level. For instance, the light setting will allow enemies to be up to four difficulty levels below the players, while the heavy setting keeps enemies at the same difficulty level as the player (Dumont, 2018). This kind of dynamic scaling has been found to be the most successful at inducing flow in-game players (Chen, 2007).

Provide Clear Feedback

Video games, such as *ACO*, give very clear and immediate feedback. This feedback may be through an avatar's virtual death, winning a race, force feedback through a controller, losing health, sound and music, visual cues, or achieving a high score; it is quite clear when you win or lose (for a more detailed discussion of feedback in video games, see Chapter 5 in this volume).

Throughout this process, the player must be actively engaged and focused on the task; otherwise, the player may quickly face a situation where there are too many enemies to defeat. In *ACO*, for example, when an enemy fort is being explored and an enemy notices you, there are a few moments where the player can choose to hide, leave the fort, or stay to fight. If the player chooses to stay, then other enemies will be notified and a call for help may go out through a signal fire, which alerts additional enemies to join the fight against the character. Being intensely focused on these visual and auditory cues enables the player to effectively proceed through the game. The integration of achievement systems also contributes to the feedback loop, letting players know how successfully they are proceeding through the game content.

Remove Distractions to Focus the Users' Attention

The merging of action and awareness occurs when the first three conditions are combined with the reduction of other distractions. For example, in *ACO*, the player effectively inhabits the character on the screen, and awareness of the video game world supersedes the real world as the player becomes immersed. This experience is vastly different from the passive experience of watching a movie or reading a book. It is also important to note that with current technology, the game worlds themselves are immersive in and of themselves. Simply wandering through the open world and enjoying its beauty can be a rewarding experience on its own, which adds to the game's level of immersion.

Due to the combination of all of these qualities, video games are adept at inducing a state of flow in-games across genre, from the casual puzzle games such as *Candy Crush* to more complicated adventure games such as *ACO*. As concisely described by Sherry (2004), video games (1) provide concrete goals and rules; (2) have actions that can be adjusted to one's capabilities; (3) provide clear feedback; and (4) remove distractions through visual and aural information to focus the users' attention. These qualities, combined with video games' accessibility and popularity, contribute to video games being an ideal space to create and maintain flow experiences (Sherry, 2004). But how does being in a state of flow translate to *learning* how to be mindful in our everyday experiences?

How Do Video Games Teach Us to Be Mindful?

Video games' ability to induce a state of flow also makes them very effective learning tools associated with mindfulness (Corcos, 2018; Csikszentmihalyi & LeFevre, 1989; Gee, 2007; Kirriemuir, 2003; Kozhevnikov, Li, Wong, Obana, & Amihai, 2018; Moneta & Csikszentmihalyi, 1996; Sherry, 2004; Sliwinski, Katsikitis, & Jones, 2015), including relaxation (Rupp, Sweetman, Sosa, Smither, & McConnell, 2017; Snodgrass, Lacy, Francois

Dengah, Fagan, & Most, 2011; Wack & Tantleff-Dunn, 2009), improved concentration (Cardoso-Leite et al., 2016; Frye, 2019; Jones, Scholes, Johnson, Katsikitis, & Carras, 2014; Rathee, Rathee, & Bhardraj, 2014), lead to improved mood and reduced stress (Huang, Wong, Yang, Chiu, & Ting, 2017; Rieger, Wulf, Kneer, Frischlich, & Bente, 2014; Rupp et al., 2017), and the development of empathy and compassion (Chen, Hanna, Manohar, & Tobias, 2018; Coyne, Warburton, Essig, & Stockdale, 2018; Shin & Ahn, 2013).

A recent study by Sliwinski and colleagues (2015) examined how mindfulness can be unintentionally trained through game design. The researchers assessed how well digital game designs align with individual aspects of mindfulness, based on the CHIME eight mindfulness factors (awareness toward inner experiences, awareness toward outer experiences, openness to experience, decentering, acceptance, relatively of thoughts and beliefs, insightful understanding, and acting with awareness). The results indicated that a variety of digital games connect with one or more of these eight factors, suggesting that playing digital games can also increase mindfulness.

There are some video games have been developed as specific tools to hone the skills associated with mindfulness. One such example is *Tenacity*, a meditative app for the iPad specifically designed to help children and teens regulate self-attention and improve mindfulness (Center for Healthy Minds: University of Wisconsin-Madison, 2019a, 2019b; Davidson, 2012; GLS Studios, 2019). The primary gameplay is as follows: with each in-breath, the player taps the screen with one finger, but on each fifth in-breath, the players must use two fingers. With each successful two-finger tap, the scenery changes creating more distractions. The more occurrences of accurate five-count sequence, the higher the score (Goleman & Davidson, 2017). In its testing phase, participants who played 20–30 minutes a day for two weeks saw "increased connectivity between the brain's executive center in the prefrontal cortex and circuitry for focused attention" (Goleman & Davidson, 2017, p. 282). Additional results revealed that participants were better able to ignore distractions in order to focus on a person's facial features after using the *Tenacity* app (Goleman & Davidson, 2017).

PLAYNE is another example, developed by Krish Shrikumar and released in 2018. *PLAYNE* starts with a barren world. As the player meditates daily, the world transforms into lush landscape, and as the game progresses, the story of *PLAYNE* is revealed through the player's interaction with a talking fox, who is the world's guardian. The goal of the game is to improve the player's sense of calmness and well-being by using the basic meditative techniques taught in the game (Gamasutra, 2018; Taylor, 2018). *PLAYNE* currently holds a 96% positive rating on Steam with comments from players who praised the game for making it easier to learn mindfulness meditation practices and reduce anxiety. One reviewer even claimed that "[the game] has changed my life" (Valve Corporation, 2019, reviews section).

Looking Ahead

While there are relatively few studies available that directly investigate the ability for video game flow states to translate to "out-of-game" mindfulness, the potential for future research is open. Given the benefits of mindfulness training, including reduced stress, depression, negative thinking, as well as improved mood and increased compassion, one can see how a person's daily life can be enhanced by learning to be mindful. Using video games as a tool—a tool that is fun, engaging, and immersive—to improve access to mindfulness training appears to be a fruitful endeavor. Another consideration is that a large part of the US population is digitally connected. As of February 2019, the Pew Research Center (2019) reports that 96% of US adults owned cell phones, and 81% owned smartphones. These high rates of adoption are most evident in the country's youngest population where adults aged 18–29 report smartphone adoption at 96% as compared to those aged 50–64 at 79% and 65+ at 53% (Pew Research Center, 2019). Once apps and games are developed to more fully incorporate all aspects of mindfulness training, this ease of access through mobile devices puts mindfulness training literally in the palm of one's hands.

References

Bergland, C. (2015, April 22). 10 ways mindfulness and meditation promote well-being. *Psychology Today*. Retrieved from https://www.psychologytoday.com/us/blog/the-athletes-way/201504/10-ways-mindfulness-and-meditation-promote-well-being.

Bowman, N. D. (2008). A PAT on the back: Media flow theory revis(it)ed. *Rocky Mountain Communication Review, 4*(1), 27–39.

Bowman, N. D., Kowert, R., & Ferguson, C. J. (2015). The impact of video game play on human (and orc) creativity. In G. P. Green & J. C. Kaufman (Eds.), *Video games and creativity*. San Diego, CA: Academic Press.

Brown, K. W., & Ryan, R. M. (2003). The benefits of being present: Mindfulness and its role in psychological well-being. *Journal of Personality and Social Psychology, 84*(4), 822–848.

Cardoso-Leite, P., Kludt, R., Vignola, G., Ma, W. J., Green, C. S., & Bavelier, D. (2016). Technology consumption and cognitive control. *Attention, Perception, & Psychophysics, 78*, 218–241. https://doi.org/10.3758/s13414-015-0988-0.

Center for Healthy Minds: University of Wisconsin-Madison. (2019a). *Dr. Richard J. Davidson*. Retrieved from https://centerhealthyminds.org/about/founder-richard-davidson.

Center for Healthy Minds: University of Wisconsin-Madison. (2019b). *Games to teach mindfulness and compassion to adolescents*. Retrieved from https://centerhealthyminds.org/science/studies/games-to-teach-mindfulness-and-compassion-to-adolescents.

Chen, A., Hanna, J. J., Manohar, A., & Tobia, A. (2018). Teaching empathy: The implementation of a video game into a psychiatry clerkship curriculum. *Academic Psychiatry: The Journal of the American Association of Directors of Psychiatric Residency Training and the Association for Academic Psychiatry, 42*(3), 362–365. https://doi.org/10.1007/s40596-017-0862-6.

Chen, J. (2007). Flow in video games (and everything else)—A well-designed game transports its players to their personal flow zones, delivering genuine feelings of pleasure and happiness. *Communications in the ACM, 50*(4), 31–34.

Corcos, A. (2018). Being enjoyably challenged is key to an enjoyable gaming experience: An experimental approach in a first-person shooter game. *Socioaffective Neuroscience & Psychology, 8*(1), 1–10. https://doi.org/10.1080/20009011.2018.1474668.

Coyne, S. M., Warburton, W. A., Essig, L. W., & Stockdale, L. A. (2018). Violent video games, externalizing behavior, and prosocial behavior: A five-year longitudinal study during adolescence. *Developmental Psychology, 54*(10), 1868–1880. https://doi.org/10.1037/dev0000574.

Csikszentmihalyi, M. (1975). *Beyond boredom and anxiety*. San Francisco, CA: Josey-Bass Publishers.

Csikszentmihalyi, M. (1990). *Flow: The psychology of optimal experience*. New York, NY: HarperCollins Publishers.

Csikszentmihalyi, M. (1993). *The evolving self*. New York, NY: Harper and Row Publishing.

Csikszentmihalyi, M., & LeFevre, J. (1989). Optimal experience in work and leisure. *Journal of Personality and Social Psychology, 56*, 815–822.

Davidson, R. (2012). Games for character and mindfulness. *The Futurist, 46*(5), 14.

Drosman, D. J. (2015). *Intrinsic motivation and well-being of runners: The role of mindfulness and flow in self-determination theory* (Doctoral dissertation). Retrieved from ProQuest Dissertations & Theses database (UMI No. 3703636).

Dumont, J. (2018). *Assassin's creed odyssey* [Video game]. Montreuil, France: Ubisoft Entertainment SA.

Frazer, C., & Stathas, S. A. (2015). Mindfulness: Being present in the moment. *International Journal of Childhood Education, 30*(2), 77–84.

Frye, D. (2019). The future of focus. *Psychology Today, 52*(2), 44–47.

Gamasutra. (2018, June 22). *PLAYNE: The meditation game launches on Steam!* Retrieved from https://www.gamasutra.com/view/pressreleases/320579/PLAYNE_The_Meditation_Game_Launches_on_Steam.php.

Gee, J. P. (2007). *What video games have to teach us about learning and literacy.* New York, NY: St. Martin's Griffin.

GLS Studios. (2019). *Projects.* Retrieved from http://glsstudios.com/games.html.

Goleman, D., & Davidson, R. (2017). *Altered traits: Science reveals how meditation changes your mind, brain, and body.* New York, NY: Avery.

Heckenberg, R. A., Hale, M. W., Kent, S., & Wright, B. J. (2019). An online mindfulness-based program is effective in improving affect, over-commitment, optimism and mucosal immunity. *Physiology & Behavior, 199*, 20–27. https://doi.org/10.1016/j.physbeh.2018.11.001.

Hoffman, C. (2010). Does mindfulness increase wellbeing? *Journal of Holistic Healthcare, 7*(1), 45–48.

Huang, H.-C., Wong, M.-K., Yang, Y.-H., Chiu, H.-Y., & Teng, C.-I. (2017). Impact of playing exergames on mood states: A randomized controlled trial. *Cyberpsychology, Behavior and Social Networking, 20*(4), 246–250. https://doi.org/10.1089/cyber.2016.0322.

Husgafvel, V. (2016). On the Buddhist roots of contemporary non-religious mindfulness practice: Moving beyond sectarian and essentialist approaches. *Temenos, 52*(1), 87–126. https://doi.org/10.1080/14639940802556560.

Ilies, R., Wagner, D., Wilson, K., Ceja, L., Johnson, M., DeRue, S., & Ilgen, D. (2017). Flow at work and basic psychological needs: Effects on well-being. *Applied Psychology: An International Review, 66*(1), 3–24. https://doi.org/10.1111/apps.12075.

Jackson, S. (2016). Flowing with mindfulness: Investigating the relationship between flow and mindfulness. In I. Ivtzan & T. Lomas (Eds.), *Mindfulness in positive psychology: The science of meditation and wellbeing* (pp. 141–155). New York, NY: Routledge/Taylor & Francis Group. https://doi.org/10.4324/9781315747217.

Jones, C. M., Scholes, L., Johnson, D., Katsikitis, M., & Carras, M. C. (2014, March 5). Gaming well: Links between video games and flourishing mental health. *Frontiers in Psychology, 5*, 1–8. https://doi.org/10.3389/fpsyg.2014.00260.

Juncaj, S. (2017). *Police officers' job satisfaction and well-being: The influences of flow* (Unpublished doctoral dissertation). Pleasantville, NY: Pace University.

Kabat-Zinn, J. (1994). *Wherever you go, there you are: Mindfulness meditation in everyday life*. New York, NY: Hyperion.

Kabat-Zinn, J. (2002). Mindfulness is about paying attention. *Reflections, 3*(3), 68–71. https://doi.org/10.1162/152417302317363949.

Kabat-Zinn, J. (2017). Mindfulness-based interventions in context: Past, present, and future. In B. A. Guadiano (Ed.), *Mindfulness: Clinical applications of mindfulness and acceptance—Specific interventions for psychiatric, behavioural, and physical health conditions* (Vol. III, pp. 363–382). New York, NY: Routledge/Taylor & Francis Group. https://doi.org/10.1093/clipsy/bpg016.

Kabat-Zinn, J. (2018). A study in healing and the mind. *Mindfulness, 9*(5), 1659–1663. https://doi.org/10.1007/s12671-018-0997-x.

Kirriemuir, J. (2003). *The relevance of video games and gaming consoles to the higher and further education learning experience*. Retrieved from https://pdfs.semanticscholar.org/e184/4c977fdef8192ce658e5cb86db18be9cec42.pdf?_ga=2.18678969.1026218792.1561412981-419805529.1558638648.

Kozhevnikov, M., Li, Y., Wong, S., Obana, T., & Amihai, I. (2018). Do enhanced states exist? Boosting cognitive capacities through an action video-game. *Cognition, 173*, 93–105. https://doi.org/10.1016/j.cognition.2018.01.006.

Martinez, C. T., & Scott, C. (2016). Trail and ultrarunning: The impact of distance, nature, and personality on flow and well-being. *Psi Chi Journal of Psychological Research, 21*(1), 6–15.

Mayo Clinic Health Systems. (2015, June 1). *Use mindfulness to improve well-being*. Retrieved from https://mayoclinichealthsystem.org/hometown-health/speaking-of-health/use-mindfulness-to-improve-well-being.

Moneta, G. B., & Csikszentmihalyi, M. (1996). The effect of perceived challenges and skills on the quality of subjective experience. *Journal of Personality, 64*(2), 275–310. https://doi.org/10.1111/j.1467-6494.1996.tb00512.x.

Nhat Hanh, T. (2017). *Thich Nhat Hanh on the practice of mindfulness*. Retrieved from https://www.lionsroar.com/mindful-living-thich-nhat-hanh-on-the-practice-of-mindfulness-march-2010/.

Pew Research Center. (2019). *Mobile fact sheet*. Retrieved from https://www.pewinternet.org/fact-sheet/mobile/.

Pickert, K. (2014, February 3). The art of being mindful: Finding peace in a stressed-out, digitally dependent culture may just be a matter of thinking differently. *Time, 183*(4), 40–46.

Rathee, N. K., Rathee, V. S., & Bhardraj, S. (2014). Concentration, reactive-proactive aggression, non-verbal aggression, and wellness among video games playing adolescents. *The International Journal of Science in Society, 5*(1), 33–41. https://doi.org/10.18848/1836-6236/cgp/v05i01/51415.

Rieger, D., Wulf, T., Kneer, J., Frischlich, L., & Bente, G. (2014). The winner takes it all: The effect of in-game success and need satisfaction on mood repair

and enjoyment. *Computers in Human Behavior, 39,* 281–286. https://doi.org/10.1016/j.chb.2014.07.037.

Rupp, M. A., Sweetman, R., Sosa, A. E., Smither, J. A., & McConnell, D. S. (2017). Searching for affective and cognitive restoration: Examining the restorative effects of casual video game play. *Human Factors, 59*(7), 1096–1107. https://doi.org/10.1177/0018720817715360.

Ryan, R. M., & Deci, E. L. (2001). On happiness and human potentials: A review of research on hedonic and eudaimonic well-being. *Annual Review of Psychology, 52*(1), 141–166. https://doi.org/10.1146/annurev.psych.52.1.141.

Sedlár, M. (2014). Relationships between flow experiences, life meaningfulness and subjective well-being in music students. *Psychology and Its Contexts, 5*(1), 89–104.

Sherry, J. L. (2004). Flow and media enjoyment. *Communication Theory, 14*(4), 328–347. https://doi.org/10.1111/j.1468-2885.2004.tb00318.x.

Shin, D.-H., & Ahn, D. (2013). Associations between game use and cognitive empathy: A cross-generational study. *Cyberpsychology, Behavior and Social Networking, 16*(8), 599–603. https://doi.org/10.1089/cyber.2012.0639.

Sliwinski, J., Katsikitis, M., & Jones, C. M. (2015). Mindful gaming: How digital games can improve mindfulness. In J. Abascal, S. Barbosa, M. Fetter, T. Gross, P. Palanque, & M. Winckler (Eds.), *Human-computer interaction—INTERACT 2015: Proceedings from the 15th IFIP TC 13 international conference* (pp. 167–184). Bamberg, Germany: Springer.

Snodgrass, J. G., Lacy, M. G., Francois Dengah, H. J. 2nd, Fagan, J., & Most, D. E. (2011). Magical flight and monstrous stress: Technologies of absorption and mental wellness in Azeroth. *Culture, Medicine and Psychiatry, 35*(1), 26–62. https://doi.org/10.1007/s11013-010-9197-4.

Taylor, H. (2018, August 17). *PLAYNE: Encouraging mindfulness through video games.* Retrieved from https://www.gamesindustry.biz/articles/2018-08-17-playne-encouraging-mindfulness-through-video-games.

Valve Corporation. (2019). *PLAYNE: The meditation game.* Retrieved from https://store.steampowered.com/app/865540/PLAYNE__The_Meditation_Game/.

Wack, E., & Tantleff-Dunn, S. (2009). Relationships between electronic game play, obesity, and psychosocial functioning in young men. *CyberPsychology & Behavior, 12*(2), 241–244. https://doi.org/10.1089/cpb.2008.0151.

Weber, R., Huskey, R., & Craighead, B. (2017). Flow experiences and well-being: A media neuroscience perspective. In L. Reinecke & M. B. Oliver (Eds.), *The Routledge handbook of media use and well-being* (pp. 183–198). New York, NY: Routledge.

White, L. B. (2014). *Mindfulness 101: Learn how living in the moment can relieve stress, improve health, and promote feelings of peace, joy and love.* Retrieved from https://www.motherearthliving.com/health-and-wellness/mind-and-body/mindfulness-present-moment-zm0z14ndzhou.

CHAPTER 8

Follow the Trail of Enemies

Emory S. Daniel Jr.

Abstract Difficult games have become a popular avenue for players who enjoy a test of skill. Gamers often like to seek challenges, break constraints within the rules of a game, and create new levels of difficulty to create a new play experience. Often though, when we find difficulty in games, the instinct is to quit playing. However, if we are persistent and change up our strategies, we are able to not only beat a boss, but also grow psychologically. The goal of this chapter is to recognize how gamers can overcome cognitive dissonance within a hard game, beat the challenge in front of them, and how that accomplishment can transfer to other activities in life.

Keywords Cognitive dissonance · Intrinsic motivators · Psychological growth

E. S. Daniel Jr. (✉)
Appalachian State University, Boone, NC, USA

R. Kowert (ed.), *Video Games and Well-being*,
Palgrave Studies in Cyberpsychology,
https://doi.org/10.1007/978-3-030-32770-5_8

> *I think most people would be better off with more pain in their lives, honestly. I think that, if nothing else, they would appreciate the pain-free times more. But I think also there's this self-induced aspect of, you've struggled, you've overcome, you've gotten through, then you're confident and you enjoy the rest of your life more, but also you feel like you can do things and you can take on challenges that you wouldn't otherwise try, and you get to points you wouldn't otherwise reach.*
> —The Barkley Marathons: The Race that Eats Its Young

What makes something difficult? Running a marathon is difficult because of the strain it puts on your body over a period of time. A PhD is difficult for the academic rigor as the constant challenges over the course of classwork, comprehensive exams, and a dissertation. Beating Super Mario Brothers 3 with no continues and no warps is hard, but there are incredibly high fail rates in certain levels in Mario Maker.

While it is incredible that there are trials specifically placed to challenge humans to push them past their absolute physical and mental capacity, it is perhaps even more fascinating that many people actively and willingly pursue difficult activities, knowing that their chance to succeed are almost none. Just as people continue to compete in ultra-marathons and pursue doctoral degrees, people seek out difficult games (Serrels, 2014). What is the secret to persisting through such difficult challenges?

This chapter will explore these questions using the lens of difficult games as an example for exploring the capacity we have as human beings have to pursue and persist through seemingly insurmountable challenges.

Seeking Out a Challenge

As video games have progressed, so has the discussion of how difficult any particular video game should be. In early generation console gaming, the hardware could only support so much content on-screen, but ultimately had to keep a player engaged for a significant period of time (Pot, 2018) This presented a conundrum for many game developers to make video games that were intentionally hard to increase run time, and thus coined the term "Nintendo Hard" (Enger, 2011). Video games such as *Contra* (KONAMI), *Battletoads* (Rare), *Super Punch Out* (Nintendo), and probably the most difficult, *PacMan* (Namco). *PacMan* was actually so difficult, it was never meant to actually be winnable. At the notorious level 256 of the game the software actually crashed and *PacMan* would end up circling around unfinished code (Hodges, 2007). At this point in time, it was rare for a game to focus on the narrative of the story, and instead focused on increasing the difficulty level and achieving a higher score.

Nowadays games have progressed past "unwinnable" and high scores to challenges supported by strong narratives, a trend that has largely garnered support from players (Melissinos, 2015). However, this has not stopped developers from continuing to incorporate high levels of difficulty. Many of new titles seem to have been created in homage to the "Nintendo Hard" generation of players, as they use similar graphics and level of difficulty, but also insert a strong narrative, gameplay, and interaction with the world to keep the player engaged (Linton, 2017). For example, games such as *Dark Souls* (FromSoftware) and *Hollow Knight* (Team Cherry) maintain a unique and engaging story but are marketed as "difficult" games.

Just as an ultra-marathon appeals to a specific athlete, the appeal of the difficulty of the game also attracts a certain demographic invested in playing games that are challenging, such as speedrunners,[1] achievement hunters,[2] or even a "hard core gamer".[3] Taking a closer look as to why people pursue these kinds of games provides insight into why we as human beings seek and persist through the various other challenges in our lives.

Challenge Seeking

Research has found several motivations for seeking and persisting through difficult in-game challenges, such constraint satisfaction (working within them or breaking them), mastery orientation, and the desire to feel a sense of achievement.

Constraint Satisfaction

Constraint satisfaction was originally developed to refer to solving a puzzle within the constraints of the parameters of a puzzle (Tsang, 2014). For

[1] Gamers whose goal is to beat a game as quickly as possible.

[2] Gamers who take achievements that are listed by the game and try to complete them.

[3] Gamers who consistently play on the toughest difficulty settings.

example, a Sudoku puzzle[4] has limited constraints to work around because of the limitations of options in the game structure and rules. Similarly, *Dark Souls* (FromSoftware, 2011) might be known for its difficulty, but the patterns of the game are primarily clear. There are parameters in which the enemy and player can move, there are boundaries in the world that the player and enemy can move in, and there are restrictions in the pattern and rhythm of the enemy's attack pattern. Thus, with practice and time, a player can adapt to the restriction and resolve a way to defeat the enemy. This is not a feat that happens within the first couple of attempts, it often takes a great deal of undertakings before a player can adapt to the enemy. Therefore, a player must be persistent within the rules and patterns of the game in order to succeed. Although there are some gamers that decide to get creative with what traditional rules indicate.

Breaking Constraints

In addition to finding success within the constraints of the rules, there are those who delight in finding ways to "break" the constraints. Some individuals thrive on completing challenges by eliminating the constraints entirely by uses of clips oversights and limitations of the challenge itself, such as the programming of a video game (Muncy, 2016). For example, *The Legend of Zelda: Ocarina of Time* is meant to be finished in 30–40 hours. However, some players have worked glitches in the game so well, that the world record as of July 2019 is 16 minutes and 58 seconds (www.speedrun.com). The speed running community has created their own rules to finish the game by breaking through the constraints of the game itself. For them, developing their own tactics to beat a difficult game makes the overcoming the obstacle that much more enjoyable.

In our day-to-day lives, individuals who are motivated by "breaking constraints" are likely those high in "sensation seeking", a personality trait reflecting a pattern to find novel, rewarding situations and stimuli, and a willingness to take risks in doing so (Zuckerman, 1994). For example, if you were in an office, engaging in a monotonous activity that was instructed for you to complete in a specific way, you might look to break that method in search of one that's more efficient. In many cases, this might be frowned upon by a supervisor as, "this is the way it's always been done" but sensation

[4] A 3 × 3 or 9 × 9 box puzzle game where boxes in every row and every column must include all numbers 1–9.

seekers would often look past that and take the risk in order to make a more enjoyable solution.

Mastery Orientation

Individuals who are self-challengers (i.e., are mastery oriented) are those who seek challenging tasks and persistence in the face of failure (Dweck & Leggett, 1988). In the context of video games, these kinds of people are often framed as "completionists" as they focus on achieving every-single intended in-game challenge (Kahn et al., 2015).

Similar to those motivated by breaking constraints, self-challengers are likely find the typical means of completing an activity becomes repetitive after a while and therefore loses excitement. If we are very good at something, we might also challenge ourselves in recreational activities to make it harder for ourselves when we get bored. For example, I consider myself an excellent skier, and so on occasion I will attempt to ski down terrain with one ski. Testing the boundaries is common among those who engage in sensation seeking activities. Supporting this notion, research has found that individuals who pursue challenges with the goal of *learning* verse the goal of *performing* are more likely to be mastery-oriented individuals (Dweck & Leggett, 1988; Elliott & Dweck, 1988).

Desire to Achieve/Salience Motivators

Salience motivators are individuals who seek out challenges out of a desire to achieve something that is otherwise unachievable (Puglisi-Allegra & Ventura, 2012). The satisfaction that is felt when doing so is reinforced by our neurochemistry as when we accomplish a difficult task, dopamine, a neurotransmitter that is known as a reward-motivated behavior, is released into our system (Berridge, Robinson, & Aldridge, 2009). If any particular challenge offers a difficult, but fair challenge that increases our likelihood to continue playing (partially because of its enabling of "flow", discussed in more detail in Chapter 1 of this volume).

While popular conversation has been linked to external incentives to maintain motivation to continue engaging (e.g., video games and loot boxes; Wiltshire, 2017) the dopamine releases can be much smaller for this kind of variable-rate reinforcement (i.e., unpredictable rewards), which can diminish motivation after a period of time (Daw & Tobler, 2014). A real-world example might be people who spend money frequently might receive small dopamine releases because of small purchases that increase their happiness. However, a person who saves up for a house might not have as much dopamine release until they buy the house, then the release is that much greater. In games and in life, difficult challenges and satisfying rewards make us want to pursue even more difficult challenges.

While these motivations explain why we seek difficult challenge, the question remains as to what threshold are we willing to endure before quitting on the challenge all together?

Cognitive Dissonance

After countless attempts at failing to overcome a trail, whether it be the Turbo Tunnel from *Battletoads* (Rare) or trying your best on a paper and not achieving the outcome you desire, it is natural to start to doubt one's abilities. This sense of doubt creates a mental discomfort, called cognitive dissonance, and for many individuals, it can make the prospect of going through the journey seem not to be worth the reward at the end.

Cognitive dissonance is a term first used by Festinger, Riecken, and Schachter (1956) in relation to how doomsday cult members would react when the world did not end. They had to reconcile a reality that conflicted with a strongly held belief. Their belief that the world would end was objectively false and now they had to reconcile why the outcome that happened did not match what they envisioned. This feeling of inconsistency is what they called cognitive dissonance which has three main components: a consonant relationship, initiation of dissonance, and unpleasant arousal (Festinger et al., 1956).

As humans, we desire consonant relationships. That is, two elements in equilibrium (Festinger, 1957). For example, if you are playing a game that was advertised as relaxing and the game is relaxing and enjoyable, then you will experience a sense of mental equilibrium because your expectations are met. However, if you are told that you would have the day off and you get called back to work, then you would experience mental disequilibrium because your expectations were not met. The dissonance occurs when the expectations experience ***disequilibrium***. This is when dissonance becomes discomforting, as we have to reconcile having two inconsistent attitudes, thoughts, beliefs, opinions, or behaviors.

Cognitive Dissonance in Practice

When I travel, I pass the time on an airplane playing video games. On a recent flight to Salt Lake City, I found myself playing a moderately hard, yet enjoyable game for myself: *The Legend of Zelda: Breath of the Wild* (BoTW). I note that the game is difficult particularly due to one enemy: The Lynel. The Lynel looks like a centaur, and deals punishing damage, has unwavering accuracy, is highly aggressive, and surprisingly fast for an enemy of its size. They are not mandatory enemies to defeat. However, it was recommended, from the story, that I get some items where this Lynel was located (e.g., shock arrows). So as I met the foe to get the arrows, and not playing this type of Zelda game before, I approached it like I would any other enemy: directly.

As expected from a challenging enemy, this strategy proved to be a fruitless endeavor as I was cut down in two strokes of the Lynel's weapon. This was my first inconsistent attitude about how this game was presented. I was still relatively new to BoTW, so my dissonance was not particularly elevated. This time, I climbed the mountain, saved the game, and proceeded to try the similar strategy with a predictable outcome. It was at this point where initiation of dissonance started to begin and an unpleasant arousal occurred almost simultaneously. I tried sneaking around the beast but had trouble with that strategy. As soon as the creature spotted me, I was done for. While my frustration was high, I had to tone it down because we were mid-flight and I was the middle seat. My first thought about this section of the game was: "Maybe I am just not good enough to beat BoTW". The only way to reduce dissonance, in my mind, was accept defeat and play something else. However, I did not have any additional games with me on my Switch. So, it was either continue on or twiddle my thumbs on the flight. Since I decided to keep playing, I was determined to find a new method to achieve consonance. So instead of continuously being beaten, I jumped off the mountain with my paraglider and attempted to approach the challenge a new way.

I searched for food to help me regain my health (thank you, durian fruits) and crafted new dishes to increase my attack, stealth, and endurance. I searched for better weapons. I found ways to upgrade my armor. And while I thought these preparations were sufficient, I was wrong. Even after all the training and obtaining supplementary items and weapons, I still could only manage to bring down the beast's health down to half. All of the work to approach things differently demonstrates that even if there is a change to remove dissonance, the inconsistency and unpleasant arousal can relapse. This time, the magnitude of dissonance had increased. Festinger (1957) addressed the concept of magnitude to the point that the dissonance has such severity; it has resulted in psychological stress that brought actual physical discomfort. From this point, I had four options of moving forward:

First, I could ignore or deny the information conflicting with the existing belief, which is to say that the Lynel was technically not necessary to beat the game. I could continue to play and completely avoid all Lynels that I see. Second, I could justify the behavior by adding new cognitions. In this case, I could go and purchase ancient arrows[5] and defeat a Lynel with one shot, eliminating the prospect of fighting them.[6,7] Third, I could justify the behavior by changing the conflicting cognition. This would be the example of me cooking and acquiring better weapons to defeat the beast. Lastly, I could change the behavior or cognition. In this case, I could either quit, or continue to press forward. So, I changed my attack strategy, while also changing my cognition that I was capable of bringing down the Lynel. I decided that I should use my bow to get a few opportunities of attack before the animal noticed me, I practiced the flurry rush[8] and timed my attacks better, I recognized patterns and was patient to take advantage of the opportunities given to me. Ultimately, after a long fight with intense focus, I emerged victorious. I wanted to cheer in jubilation, but I remembered that I was elbow to elbow with two strangers and they might not appreciate my gesture of victory.

The story illustrates the complexity of the cognitive dissonance by demonstrating that we experience a sense of greater value when overcoming a difficult challenge. As it turns out, every other enemy in the game paled in comparison to the difficulty of the Lynel. Every subsequent boss felt like a small challenge at worst, to a cakewalk at best. Overcoming that challenge made me feel like I could conquer any upcoming encounter that was presented. That feeling was euphoric, I achieved cognitive consonance

[5] Which are rare, highly expensive, and should ideally be saved for very specific situations.

[6] Which, admittedly, was how the author fought most Lynels when he didn't want to put in the time or the resources to beat the creature in the traditional manner.

[7] If you shoot the Lynel with the ancient arrow, you eliminate the beast, but you also do not receive any rewards for doing so. It's a tradeoff for those who are akin to adding a new cognition.

[8] A slow motion, frame perfect dodge, that narrowly escapes an attack and allows the player several hits in without interference from the enemy.

about overcoming this problem, and the overall outcome was that I grew in understanding the game (and I was able to reap the in-game rewards associated with my success).

Another example of overcoming cognitive dissonance could be drawn from my graduate school experience. Graduate school is a very difficult process, and as a person progresses through it, most individuals experience a dissonance in whether or not they can succeed in earning an advanced degree. As the challenges pile on, they may feel like they cannot proceed any longer for a myriad of reasons. Which means that they might change their cognition to say that they didn't need graduate school. Whereas if I take my lessons from the Lynel and apply it to graduate school, maybe my cognition should be more focused on changing my behavior entirely. Maybe I should study differently, seek other means of support, reinvent my writing, which ultimately can lead to a positive change. What is important is that we realize we *can* do it, and it could be that any small success is the spark for more motivation to persist.

Benefits of Being Persistent

Persisting in the face of challenges can impact more than just the immediate sense of accomplishment. Practicing persistence and pushing through challenges to success can lead to other short- and long-term psychological benefits.

Cognitive Consonance

The immediate result of accomplishment will provide a sense of cognitive consonance, or mental stability. After the struggle of fighting the Lynel my feelings of dissonance dissipated as the question of "can I defeat this challenge" was answered with a resounding yes. Individuals can achieve this sense of consonance by failing at beating the boss and thus declaring that they do not need to beat it or by defeating the boss and answering the aforementioned question by determining "yes I can defeat the challenge". Consonance is a state of harmony and internal consistency that is compatible with one's previous attitudes (Festinger, 1957). With the BoTW example, if I lose enough times, I might feel deflated and change my cognition completely (e.g., I don't need to beat this enemy or this game is too hard). Conversely, if I continue to master my abilities and push through the struggle, I will also achieve an internal consistency. Except this time, I will look into how I can expand my abilities, explore new challenges, and redefine my abilities. This is an essential and powerful process, as now we are redefining our preconceived notions of we are capable of (Harmon-Jones, 2002). After I defeated the Lynel, I felt like I could take on any enemy. This exploration and re-appropriation transcends past my initial success into other areas of growth and learning.

Psychological Growth

As humans we strive to satisfy needs and exceed them as we reach different stages of their life. Merton (1948) coined the term "self-fulfilling prophecy" as a prediction about oneself that becomes true, often resulting from positive feedback between the belief and behavior. If people are positively progressing and working to exceed expectations, the actions and desires of the person often match what their beliefs are beforehand which can lead to some positive outcomes of growth. The success achieved can be aspirational material for oneself to embracing higher values and ideals for oneself. Beating a difficult boss in is gratifying, and it can make players consider what else they could accomplish because of those increased values.

Growth also means self-awareness, which can help a person to discover their own personalities and how they can better change them, which in turn helps us create better understanding of others. Often discussed under the umbrella of social comparison theory (Festinger, 1954), this means that we look for comparisons from other people's abilities and talents. While watching twitch streams of professional gamers, viewers will observe for the same reason a child watches a professional athlete, to personally get better. As community members make upward comparisons, some positive effects can lead to hope and inspiration to do better themselves (Tesser, 1988). One of the long-term outcome of overcoming dissonance is this kind of positive psychological growth, such as greater joy in personal accomplishments of oneself and others (Tajfel & Turner, 1979), increased self-efficacy, personal expectations, and self-awareness (Baumeister, 2010; Steele & Liu, 1983; Wigfield, Guthrie, Tonks, & Perencevich, 2004), and changes in individuality (Reiss, 2004).

The organizer of the Barkley Marathons (arguably one of the most difficult ultra-marathons in the world) stated that many of the participants that wanted the challenge and conquered the challenge were adventurers or graduate students. Within the context of cognitive dissonance and consonance this makes sense—those who accomplish earning a graduate degree are likely to continue to seek and find challenges to overcome.

Similarly, for those who played *Guitar Hero 3: Legends of Rock* (Neversoft), the most difficult challenge in the entire game was completing "Through the Fire and the Flames" by Dragonforce on expert mode. Those who were able to accomplish this feat of dexterity, achieved consonance and enjoyed a nice dopamine release for motivation. However, maybe the challenge did not end with that level or even the game, maybe a person fresh off their victory can recognize the time and effort put into that challenge and can consider that maybe they could apply that commitment to other areas of their life.

This could mean taking greater joy in personal accomplishments and others' accomplishments as well. For example, many speed running communities pride their involvement in their community as a positive, nurturing, and supportive atmosphere. Stating on many occasions at *Games Done Quick* (GDQ) they enjoy seeing their friends in the community succeed even though they are competing against each other for the fastest time.[9] Psychologists describe the level of involvement and commitment to a group had a strong impact in one's overall conceptualization of self (Tajfel & Turner, 1979). Social identity theory (Tajfel & Turner, 1979) explains how people enjoy being part of a greater group, in which all members[10] can bond over each other's joy for a game. Thus, being able to become more positive toward other people's accomplishments. Belonging to a group with strong identity will more often encourage collaboration and celebration for members' victories because they participate in the same community. Understanding a gamer is part of an elite group of skilled players creates that positivity for themselves and for others.

Another positive outcome could be increased self-awareness, self-efficacy, and personal expectations (Baumeister, 2010; Steele & Liu, 1983; Wigfield, et al. 2004). Players might begin to feel more self-reliant after defeating a difficult boss without needing the help of others. Critically thinking to best way to solve a problem or creating unorthodox thinking contributes to self-sufficiency. Although this will not always occur, achieving success is often a first step in increasing values.

Lastly, there can be changes in personal beliefs and attitudes, sometimes referred to as individuality (Reiss, 2004). As mentioned with cognitive

[9] Personal favorite example of competitiveness and community is Md_Neo vs. KVD in the Super Mario Kart Race https://www.youtube.com/watch?v=q7JTayEh4SY.

[10] With varying degrees of experience and involvement.

dissonance, much of our dissonance resides in an inconsistency of personal attitudes. As people achieve consonance, they will often re-examine those beliefs and attitudes and might discover something about themselves that might give them a sense of pride. For example, as a child, I rented NBA Jam (Midway Games) from a video store and was close to beating the game by defeating all NBA teams in a career mode. Unfortunately, I had to turn the game back into the store. However, I went with my father to the video store and he asked me "how many more teams did you have to beat", I told him only five. As a way to teach me an unorthodox life lesson, my father did not turn in the game, but instead extended the rental and watched me beat the remaining five teams. Teaching the value of finishing what you started was very important to him, and it became a very paramount value in my individuality as well.

Intrinsic Motivators

After a while, an advantage of intrinsic motivators can lead actually lead to people moving away from this kind of motivational salience (Deci & Ryan, 1985). This is, they may become less motivated less by the goal and more driven by engaging in the activity itself (Puglisi-Allegra & Ventura, 2012). For example, Ryan & Deci (2000) found that when it came to smoking, eventually people enjoyed the task of not participating in the behavior more than the external pressures or a desire for consideration. The enjoyment comes from engaging or not engaging in the behavior rather than social influence of doing something. Simply stated, gamers might enjoy playing *Dark Souls* (FromSoftware) because they actually enjoy the difficulty. After a while, the reward of beating a boss is actually secondary, instead outcomes that follow are increased autonomy, self-efficacy, and an interest in mastery (Wigfield et al, 2004). Simply put, we are comfortable to complete tasks on our own, we feel good about the skills we have to achieve goals, and we are genuinely interested in a topic, rather than just going through the motions. Gaming can teach us this skill as we can genuinely enjoy a challenge, and the confidence gained from mastery can translate into other areas of their lives.

The Takeaway

Gaming for many is a way to relax, escape, and enjoy an activity with friends. However, for others, gaming is an opportunity to challenge their limits, and improve upon their skills. In this sense, video games are tools. While they are rarely causal in changing or reinforcing behavior, at the right moment in a person's life they can be used as a catalyst for impactful turning points. Understanding consonance in defeat and rage quitting or giving up can be a traumatic experience for some. However, it can just as easily be a tool to understand limits, how to fail, and reinvent ourselves. Overcoming dissonance in a triumphant manner might be a tool for arrogant and toxic behavior in chat. However, it can just as easily be a tool for someone struggling with self-esteem to gain confidence and overcome other obstacles. While gaming is a tool, or a catalyst, if they are used correctly and promoted as tools of transference, there are very few things that gamers cannot accomplish.

References

Battletoads [Computer Software]. (1991). Twycross, Rare.

Baumeister, R. F. (2010). The self. In E. J. Finkel & R. F. Baumeister (Eds.), *Handbook of social psychology*. New York: Oxford University Press.

Berridge, K., Robinson, T., & Aldridge, J. W. (2009). Dissecting components of reward: 'liking', 'wanting', and learning. *Current Opinion in Pharmacology, 9*(1), 65–73.

Contra [Computer Software]. (1987). Tokyo: Konami.

Dark Souls [Computer Software]. (2011). Tokyo, FromSoftware.

Daw, N. D., & Tobler, P. N. (2014). Value learning through reinforcement: The basics of dopamine and reinforcement in learning. In P. W. Glimcher & E. Fehr (Eds.), *Neuroeconomics: Decision making and the brain* (pp. 283–298). New York: Academic Press.

Deci, E. L., & Ryan, R. M. (1985). *Intrinsic motivation and self-determination in human behavior*. New York: Plenum.

Dweck, C. S., & Leggett, E. L. (1988). A social-cognitive approach to motivation and personality. *Psychological Review, 95*(2), 256–273.

Elliott, E. S., & Dweck, C. S. (1988). Goals: An approach to motivation and achievement. *Journal of Personality and Social Psychology, 54*, 5–12.

Enger, M. (2011). *What is "Nintendo hard"?* Bits 'n' Bites. https://web.archive.org/web/20110223221444/; http://bnbgaming.com/2011/02/08/what-is-nintendo-hard/.

Festinger, L. (1954). A theory of social comparison processes. *Human Relations, 7*(2), 117–140.

Festinger, L. (1957). *A theory of cognitive dissonance*. Palo Alto, CA: Stanford University Press.

Festinger, L., Riecken, H. W., & Schachter, S. (1956). *When prophecy fails*. Minneapolis, MN: University of Minnesota Press.

Guitar Hero 3: Legends of Rock [Computer Software]. (2007). Woodland Hills, Neversoft.

Harmon-Jones, E. (2002). A cognitive dissonance theory perspective on persuasion. In J. P. Dillard & M. Pfau (Eds.), *The persuasion handbook: Developments in theory and practice* (p. 1). Thousand Oaks, CA: Sage.

Hodges, D. (2007). *Splitting apart the split screen: The journey to find, analyze, and fix Pac Man's split screen*. DonHodges.com. http://www.donhodges.com/how_high_can_you_get2.htm.

Hollow Knight [Computer Software]. (2018). Adelaide, Team Cherry.

Iltis, A., & Kayne, T. J. (Producers & Directors). (2014). The Barkley Marathons: The Race That Eats Its Young [Motion Picture]. Los Angeles, USA.

Kahn, A. S., Shen, C., Lu, L., Ratan, R. A., Coary, S., Hou, J., … Williams, D. (2015). The Trojan Player Typology: A cross-genre, cross-cultural, behaviorally validated scale of video game play motivations. *Computers in Human Behavior, 49*, 354–361.

Legend of Zelda: Breath of the Wild [Computer Software]. (2017). Kyoto, Nintendo.

Linton, M. (2017). *The rise of pixel art*. Morgan Linton Blog. https://morganlinton.com/the-rise-of-pixel-art/.

Melissinos, C. (2015). Video games are one of the most important art forms in history. *Time Magazine*. http://time.com/collection-post/4038820/chris-melissinos-are-video-games-art/.

Merton, R. (1948). The self-fulfilling prophecy. *The Antioch Review, 8*(2), 195.

Muncy, J. (2016). Why videogame speedruns are so fascinating to watch. *Wired*. https://www.wired.com/2016/01/speedruns/.

NBA Jam [Computer Software]. (1993). Chicago, Midway.

PacMan [Computer Software]. (1980). Tokyo, Namco.

Pot, J. (2018). *Why old Nintendo games were so hard: The unofficial history of Nintendo hard*. How-To Geek. https://www.howtogeek.com/219142/why-old-video-games-were-so-hard-the-unofficial-history-of-nintendo-hard/.

Puglisi-Allegra, S., & Ventura, R. (2012). Prefrontal/accumbal catecholamine system processes high motivational salience. *Frontiers in Behavioral Neuroscience, 27*, https://doi.org/10.3389/fnbeh.2012.00031.

Reiss, S. (2004). Multifaceted nature of intrinsic motivation: The theory of 16 basic desires. *Review of General Psychology, 8*(3), 179–193.

Ryan, R., & Deci, E. (2000). Self-determination theory and the facilitation of intrinsic motivation, social development, and well-being. *American Psychologist, 55*(1), 68–78.

Serrels, M. (2014). *Why the Hell do we keep playing difficult video games?* Kotaku. https://kotaku.com/why-the-hell-do-we-keep-playing-difficult-video-games-1572252868.

Speedrun.com. (2019). The Legend of Zelda Ocarina of Time Any% Speedrun. https://www.speedrun.com/oot.

Steele, C. M., & Liu, T. J. (1983). Dissonance processes as self-affirmation. *Journal of Personality and Social Psychology, 45*(1), 5–19.

Super Punch Out [Computer Software]. (1994). Kyoto, Nintendo.

Tajfel, H., & Turner, J. C. (1979). An integrative theory of intergroup conflict. *The Social Psychology of Intergroup Relations, 33*, 47.

Tesser, A. (1988). Toward a self-evaluation maintenance model of social behavior. In L. Berkowitz (Ed.), *Advances in experimental social psychology, Vol. 21. Social psychological studies of the self: Perspectives and programs* (pp. 181–227). San Diego, CA: Academic Press.

Tsang, E. (2014). *Foundations of constraint satisfaction: The classic text.* Books on Demand (BOD). ISBN 978-3-7357-2366-6.

Wigfield, A., Guthrie, J., Tonks, S., & Perencevich, K. (2004). Children's motivation for reading: Domain specificity and instructional influences. *The Journal of Educational Research, 97*(6), 300–309.

Wiltshire, A. (2017). Behind the addictive psychology and seductive art of loot boxes. *PCGamer*. https://www.pcgamer.com/behind-the-addictive-psychology-and-seductive-art-of-loot-boxes/.

Zuckerman, M. (1994). *Behavioral expressions and biosocial bases of sensation seeking*. New York, NY: Cambridge University Press.

CHAPTER 9

You Are the One Foretold; Finding Yourself Through the Journey

Megan Connell and Kelli Dunlap

Abstract Through play we explore and learn about the world. The Monolith, or better known as the Hero's Journey, is a form of story in which the hero ventures out into the world to adventure, and they grow, change and learn as a result of their journey. In this chapter, we explore why digital games are such a powerful medium for expressing The Hero's Journey and explore the transformative potential of RPGs as a vehicle for personal growth and wellness.

Keywords Roleplaying games · RPG · The Hero's Journey · Avatarism · Growth mindset

M. Connell (✉)
Southeast Psych, Charlotte, NC, USA
e-mail: mconnell@southeastpsych.com

K. Dunlap
American University, Rockville, MD, USA

R. Kowert (ed.), *Video Games and Well-being*,
Palgrave Studies in Cyberpsychology,
https://doi.org/10.1007/978-3-030-32770-5_9

Play is thought by many to be fundamental to growth and development throughout the lifespan. During childhood, play is how we learn about and explore the world. It is critical for developing and practicing social skills, fostering human connection, and plays (pun intended!) an important role in shaping personal and cultural identity (Bowman, 2010). However, play is also often viewed as only appropriate for children and frivolous or childish for adults. As we grow older, play becomes devalued and the avenues through which we can play become limited with work, productivity, and being "serious" taking its place (Deterding, 2018). This is because play is often thought of as the opposite of work, which is what adults "should" be focusing all their time and energy on. However, the opposite of work is not play, it's depression (Sutton-Smith, 1997), and as such, denying play and playful expression in adulthood can have significant negative consequences to health and well-being.

In modern societies, adolescent and adult play-drives are often channeled through games. Unlike the unstructured, free-form, and autotelic (i.e., done for its own sake) play of childhood, a game is a structured play experience. For example, there's no wrong way to *play* with a baseball—you can roll it, throw it, kick it, etc. But the *game* of baseball has a lengthy list of rules that govern the play experience. This kind of play is more socially acceptable for adolescents and adults, particularly in the case with sports-based games, as they tap into the value placed on adult activities being productive (e.g., sports can improve one's health, stamina, and teamwork capabilities, etc.).

Despite the similar structure in sports-based games and video games, the perceptions of their productivity or functionality are quite different. Playing video games for recreation (i.e., playing to relax, socialize, have fun, etc.) is often held in a category separate from the other kinds of games we revere (i.e., chess, American football, the Olympics). This is, at least partially, because playing video games is frequently associated with childishness and frivolity—a hedonistic and self-indulgent pastime for the immature, socially awkward, or reclusive (Deterding, 2018; Kowert, Griffiths, & Oldmeadow, 2012). This persistent and unfortunate perception disregards video games as a play space that empowers players to do things they could never achieve otherwise. Not everyone can be an Olympic athlete, but everyone can pick up a controller and gain a sense of accomplishment, success, and meaning, things our adult lives often lack.[1]

This chapter explores how digital role-playing games can improve our psychological well-being by fostering growth, resilience, and meaningful connection. Specifically, it maps the experience of transformation through role-playing games (RPGs) to the format and structure of the Hero's Journey, a classic literary template for character transformation. The function and impact of the Hero's Journey in RPGs is compared to traditional forms of storytelling with the goal of better understanding how games can be used to support and promote psychological wellness. Key to this discussion is exploring what we gain through play due to the unique affordances of digital RPGs. The current state of research on how playing digital role-playing games impact players, the future of digital RPGs, and next steps for researchers is highlighted.

The Hero's Journey

The Hero's Journey (tHJ), also referred to as the Monomyth (Campbell, 2008), is a well-known narrative structure that centers on modeling personal growth in the face of adversity. The transformational journey takes place through three distinct acts: Departure, Initiation, and Return. In act one, *Departure*, the protagonist leaves the ordinariness of their daily life behind as they reluctantly heed the call of adventure. In act two, *Initiation*, the hero undergoes a series of trials and eventually takes on and defeats the main antagonist. In act three, *Return*, the hero returns to the ordinary world and delivers an item or piece of knowledge obtained from defeating the big bad (villain, world, natural disasters, etc.) and ultimately realizes they have been changed or transformed by their journey. This structure can be found across many forms of storytelling including film, books, and video games (Lawson, 2005).

While tHJ in film and literature has been extensively studied, the examination of video games through tHJ lens is relatively new. This is largely in part to video games being a (comparatively) newer form of narrative expression and, at least in part, to the popular perception of video games as a frivolous or dangerous form of recreation.

[1] This especially true for persons who have a physical disability as games have become increasingly accessible, i.e. color-blind mode, button-mapping, the Xbox Adaptive Controller.

Similar to other forms of media such as literature and film, games can be—and are—critically read and interpreted as texts. For example, educator Paul Darvasi integrated the video game *What Remains of Edith Finch* (Giant Sparrow, 2017) into his high school ELA curriculum and leveraged the game's themes and content as the foundation for a social and emotional learning module around identity (Darvasi, Farber, & Rivers, 2019). There is a rapidly growing population of educators using games in the classroom to engage students in content that is often unengaging or difficult to teach within the constraints of a classroom.

However, even though games can be read as texts, it is important to note that they are distinctive from other forms of media in their demand for engagement. Whereas film and books are largely passive experiences, games require active engagement from players in order for the narrative to progress. Games are also the only medium where the consumer identifies *as* the main character; the actions of the narrative are owned by the player which is why, when describing play, players use personal pronouns to describe actions rather than third-person (e.g., "I traveled to Mordor and cast the ring into Mount Doom" versus "Frodo took the ring to Mordor and cast the ring into Mount Doom"). Put another way: Readers read, viewers watch, gamers do (Grace, Dunlap, Datu, & Rice, 2016).

This distinction is important as playing through tHJ actively engages the player to take part and make decisions in a story arc that is transformational by definition and by design. This kind of active role-playing allows players to see and experience the world in a way where their choices matter, no challenge is impossible, and victory is something attainable and earned through their own knowledge, skills, and abilities. Traditional means of experiencing the Hero's Journey, such as television and film, can tell a story of growth that is received by the viewer, but in games players act out the journey and practice skills relevant to enacting a similar journey in their own lives (e.g., persistence, curiosity, problem-solving, resilience, etc.). For example, when viewing the film 12 Monkeys (1995) we can understand the bizarre ending and think about it for a time, the difficult choices James Cole had to make and the challenges he faced. It is quite another thing to spend sometimes hundreds of hours playing with a character diving deep in the dungeon to face the great evil corrupting the land, only to realize the only way to save the world is to sacrifice your character as you have to in *Diablo* (Blizzard Entertainment, 1996). For example, in the movie Spiderman Homecoming (2017), we learn that the primary villain Adrian Toomes had good reasons to start doing what he did. He wanted to provide work for his employees and a life for his family. He started taking darker and darker turns as the film progressed, yet we could understand how he got started on this road. Compare this with the gameplay experience of *Ori and the Blind Forest* (Moon Studios, 2015), an award-winning platform-adventure video game. Ori is a small forest spirit trying to make their way home while being pursued by a great angry owl. As the story unfolds, the player learns that the owl is hunting you not because they are evil but because of the traumatic loss of her owlets. She is a mother filled with rage and grief and this revelation creates a beautiful, jarring moment where the enemy transitions from a representation of evil into a being worthy of understanding, empathy, and compassion.

The interactive and immersive quality of gaming worlds provide opportunities for players to explore tHJ as a path for growth or transformation. The very nature of video games allows for a more intimate connection to the Hero's Journey because of the players' active, emotional participation in the story rather than simply emotionally identifying with the monomyth (Wrisinger, 2014).[2]

Hero's Journey—Act 1: Departure

In the traditional Hero's Journey, the *Departure* serves as a way to get to know a character and understand their perspective of the world. The tension that fuels the reluctance of the character (and consequently, the player) to depart stems from an understanding of what the protagonist is giving up by leaving and what they would be risking by refusing the call. Typically, this is a very difficult decision.

The purpose of the *Departure* phase is to get readers or viewers to care about the protagonist and what comes next. While the goals of Act 1 in an RPG is similar to that of the tHJ, the structure is markedly different. Most tHJ stories begin with the protagonist going through the rhythms of daily life. For example, in the beginning of *The Elder Scrolls V: Skyrim* (Bethesda Game Studios, 2011) your character awakens in a cart, with no knowledge of how they got there bound with other prisoners. You are led into a fort and learn that your character is to be executed. As you approach, a dragon attacks the fort and suddenly you are thrown into a scenario of running for

[2] Some examples of games that exemplify the traditional Hero's Journey include The Last of Us (Naughty Dog, 2013), Legend of Zelda: Breath of the Wild (Nintendo, 2017), and Celeste (Matt Makes Games, 2018).

your life. This is followed by a narrative hook or event to capture interest by creating conflict and setting up the protagonist to go on their quest.

When developing a game thinking about the *Departure* is important. It helps the player care about the world. Having a rich world and well-framed Act 1 is not necessary for a game to be successful, but a solid setup for the Hero's Journey helps to bring us back time and again into a gaming world. This set up is not just about creating a platform for your game, it's about setting up for your franchise. Perhaps the franchise that has done this the best is *The Legend of Zelda* (Nintendo, 1986). The characters, the myth, and the land have all been so richly developed that players care and want to return to Hyrule again, and again, and again. A good set up can lead to a strong identity with the character. The player wants to return to Hyrule again, in part because it is familiar, in part because the story is rich, and in part because they again get to be the hero of ages.

The first *Legend of Zelda* game was released in 1986 and each subsequent game has built upon the lore and the world. This allows for players to engage in a world that is familiar with well-known and often beloved NPC's a lore that they are familiar with. Having this sense of familiarity allows for a faster onboarding process for players. We know what elements will be in the story and likely what the adventure will be consist of.

Immersing ourselves in a game often results in a wide range of emotions we typically do not experience in daily life. On the pleasant side, being immersed in a game can lead to feelings such as joy, accomplishment, and pride derived from a gameplay-induced sense of mastery, self-determination, competence, and self-efficacy (McGonigal, 2015; Ryan, Rigby, & Przybylski, 2006). One rarely gets to ride a dragon or explore a lost temple on their way to work. On the unpleasant side of things, games can make us feel incompetent, frustrated, sad, fearful, and guilty. These are feelings we typically avoid whenever possible but in games, as well as other forms of art, we often seek them out. Games provide a space where we can sit with unpleasant or uncomfortable emotions and practice feeling and resolving those emotions. In other words, games enable us to more fully experience the full range of human emotion (Dunlap, 2019). And, therapeutically speaking, becoming aware of one's own emotions and the situations that evoke them is central emotion recognition and regulation, and therefore, essential for overall health and well-being (DeSteno, Gross, & Kubzansky, 2013).

It is important to note that most often tHJ occur in the context of role-playing games like *Legend of Zelda*. As such, the individual contributions of the unique features of RPGs need to be considered in relation to their potential impact on players' well-being through the use of avatars, skill-building mechanics, and immersion. Each of these elements is also individually associated with learning and personal growth. Each of these components is more briefly discussed in more detail below.

Avatars

Typically, Act 1 in RPGs are focused on getting to know the player-character, non-player characters, and the world around them. RPGs amplify the connection between player and protagonist on tHJ because the player ***is*** the protagonist. This early connection with the game is what can help to strengthen the player's bond with the world of the game, the story and the other characters.

Many, although not all, RPGs start with players creating or customizing their avatar, a representation of the player in the game-world. After this point (if required), RPGs tend to start gameplay at the tail end Act 1. During this time, RPGS introduce both the "rabbit-hole" moment and the rules of the game-world with the former typically guiding the later. A rabbit-hole moment is an element that draws the player into the fiction of the game and is often used as a way to communicate the rules, mechanics, and logics of the game (Jagoda, Gilliam, McDonald, & Russell, 2015). This often begins as narrative cutscene where the player is oriented to the game-world and is then given direct (e.g., verbal or written prompts) or indirect prompts (e.g., a path cut through the grass) on how to physically control their player-character in the digital space. Some games, such as *Witcher III* (CD Projekt, 2015), have a series of simple challenges the player-character must overcome to get from point A to point B. Other games, such as *The Elder Scrolls V: Skyrim* (Bethesda Game Studios, 2011), teach required skills during a high stakes set piece where learning the controls helps to ensure your character's survival and launches them on their journey. Because the player is often learning the same thing as their avatar (how to fight a dragon, for example) and experiencing the same emotional experiences as the avatar (wanting to slay said dragon), the player enters the game as an active and essential element of the world.

Players who create or customize their avatars, especially their avatar's cosmetic appearance, express a much stronger sense of identification with their player-character compared to players who do not have that opportunity (Turkay & Kinzer, 2014). Often the avatar can be seen as representing an idealized version of ourselves (Christy & Fox, 2016; Ducheneaut, Wen, Yee, & Wadley, 2009; Pringle 2015). By actively engaging in the game-world and interacting with others via our aspirational self, players can begin to explore their identities and, perhaps, see themselves as being more like their aspirational self (Frasca, 2003; Gee, 2003; Klimmt, Hefner, & Vorderer, 2009; Przybylski, Weinstein, Murayama, Lynch, & Ryan, 2012). In fact, research has found that our "real-world" identities continually inform the virtual identities of our avatars and vise versa (Waggoner, 2009).

This effect has been noted in literature for quite some time. For example, a 2011 study by Gabriel and Young asked participants to categorize words into "me" and "not me" words. Participants were then asked to read a passage from a *Harry Potter* book and recategorize the "me" and "not me" words. Following the readings, the participants rated more words associated with being a wizard (e.g., want, broomstick potions) as "me" rather than "not me" words. This research highlights the power of storytelling.

By engaging in a game-world as an idealized version of ourselves, or as a hero that might be nothing like us (e.g., Link in any of the *Legend of Zelda* games [Nintendo], or Master Chief in the *Halo* series [Microsoft]) can positively shift our self-perceptions to be more congruent with our idealized avatars (Frasca, 2003; Gee, 2003; Klimmt et al., 2009; Przybylski et al., 2012). Our character acted heroically or stuck with a challenge and came out the better for it, and therefore so can we (and in the game, we did!).

Skill-Building

Once the player has invested themselves in the game through the creation and customization of their avatar, they need to learn how to do... everything. RPGs also often expose players to a skill-building or tutorial content required to set off on their journey. One tool often used as a way to foster learning in games is called flow. First defined by psychologist Csikszentmihalyi (1975), flow is a psychological state of full engagement where an activity is sufficiently challenging but not too challenging. This kind of engagement is considered optimal for learning because it is the sweet spot between frustration and boredom (for more on this, see Chapter 1 in this volume). Flow states can happen with any activity, from playing sports to writing papers, but games are uniquely designed to make achieving this meaningful psychological state almost on demand.

When in a state of flow, players become hyperfocused, experience a distortion of time and space, and are often driven to continue playing because they are having a good time. These unique qualities of flow encourage learning and skill-building because players are hyperfocused and determined to complete the difficult (but not impossible) in-game challenges (Sherry, 2004).

Many games are designed to encourage flow from the very beginning of the game play experience. For example, the process of "onboarding" (i.e., introducting players to the gaming space and controls) is often designed in a way that encourages flow to rapidly build competence, confidence, and curiosity (Hodent, 2017). A good example of this comes from the game *Journey* (That Gaming Company, 2012). In this gaming space, players learn how the world works through exploration. They are given simple instructions (such as hold down a button) and nothing more and must learn how to use abilities to navigate through the world.

Video games also moderate the levels of flow through the use of dynamic difficulty settings (i.e., easy, normal, hard). That is, many video game adjust their difficulty based on player performance. A prime example of this can be seen in *Mario Kart* (Nintendo, 1992), a racing game based on Nintendo's flagship Mario franchise. *Mario Kart* uses a rubber-banding technique of non-player characters (NPCs), meaning that the better the player performs, the more challenging the NPCs perform.

These qualities combined encourage skill-building by allowing players to feel challenged but not overwhelmed, an ideal mental state for learning, practicing persistence, and producing satisfying win-states (Blasko, Lum, White, & Drabik, 2014). Put another way, it helps encourage competence and autonomy through learning, both of which are tied to greater psychological well-being (Deci & Ryan, 2008).

Story Immersion

The third component in RPGs is story immersion. Player investment in the character through the customization of an avatar and skill-building via play mechanics are not on their own to maintain players' engagement. The player also needs a story and a world that they care about. There are several techniques that can be used to drive this engagement. For example, the desire for survival. For example, in *Dragon Age: Inquisition* (Bioware, 2014) your character is blamed for an attack and is charged with helping to stop what is happening to help clear their name. In *The Elder Scrolls V: Skyrim* your character is trying to flee both their execution and a dragon attack. Another method is to present a mystery to the player. For example in *Legend of Zelda: Breath of the Wild* (Nintendo, 2017), your character awakens with no memory in a world that is full of ruins and strange large machines. You don't understand what happened and your natural curiosity can drive you to explore more and more in the world. You are rewarded with small bits of information that often lead to more questions and drive the player further into the story.

Act 2: Initiation

In the tHJ, *Initiation* is the rising action of the text. Challenges get harder, the consequences more dire, and feelings like anxiety, hopelessness, or fear begin to heighten. For most RPGs, Act 2 is going to be the bulk of the game. This is where the avatar explores the world, learns new skills, gathers loot, learns about the lands around them, solves problems, and overcomes challenges. Getting through Act 2 is difficult and can take hundreds of hours. Act 2 is about persistence.

Persistence has been shown to be a strong predictor of success (Dweck, 2007). In our daily lives failure can often come with a price, whether it be lower grades, not meeting a deadline, or disappointing our friends. In games, we can fail with fewer consequences. We get to see what happens by making mistakes, and, through persistence, eventually experience the "epic win" (McGonigal, 2010). A term coined by Jane McGonigal (2010), the epic win is when we overcome odds that we thought were insurmountable to achieve a victory bigger than we could imagine. These wins are the result of hours and hours of work. By learning about and developing the skills related to the power of persistence through video games, we can learn about and develop persistence for our daily lives.

The *Initaiation* phase of the journey can be delivered in a few different ways, it can either be an "on rails" story where player follows a set gameplay path, such as in Diablo II (Blizzard), a semi-structured adventure such as *Elder Scrolls V: Skyrim*, or *Legend of Zelda: Breath of the Wild*, or a fully open world such as *Neverwinter* (Cryptic Studios, 2016) or *World of Warcraft* (Blizzard, 2004).

In this phase, persistence is uniquely modeled in games through enthusiastic failure. To enthusiastically fail is to enthusiastically run head-long into situations where you will almost surely, repeatedly fail. Games are the art of failure; they create a space where failure is not only ok but is expected, celebrated, and designed as an opportunity to learn and try again (Juul, 2013). Think about it. How would life be different if all the times we failed learning something new, trying something different, we were met with support, guidance, and endless opportunities to try again? This is another unique feature of video games as an interactive medium—you can't fail a book or a film, but you definitely can fail a game. In fact, players are failing in one way or another 80% of the time during gameplay (e.g., falling off a cliff, losing to a difficult enemy; Lazzaro, 2004).

For example, in *Diablo II* (Blizzard North, 2000) whenever your character dies on a mission, the player is given a new avatar and the opportunity to retrieve the items from your past self, thus taking the sting of loss or regret out of failing. However, while you could recover your items, you also had to confront the enemy that previously defeated you. This gave you the chance to try, fail, try again, fail and learn.

The model of try, fail and try again was brought to new extremes with *Dark Souls* (FromSoftware, 2011) and *Sekiro: Shadows Die Twice* (FromSoftware, 2019). Both of these games were designed to challenge highly experienced gamers. You are rewarded for persistence, and trying again, and again. You do not start off powerful, you have to grind away at level after level before finally being rewarded with hard won victories. These games demonstrate the power of persistence because the only way to ever truly fail a game is to quit.

Failure is yet another way games contribute to creating a Hero's Journey experience unlike any other medium. In games, the player is responsible for the failure of the journey—failure to save the princess, failure to hop across a busy street, failure to save the human race—and the sense of ownership and complicity involved in being the cause of tragedy or suffering is a fundamental difference between games and other forms of storytelling. In games we actively live—rather than passively watch—the hero's journey, hardship, failure, and all. And maybe sometimes we triumph, which brings us to Act 3.

Act 3: The Return

In most films and books the *Return* this when the hero has finished their main quest and returns home. They find that they have changed and no longer fit into the world the way they once did. In video games this is perhaps the part that stands out the most as a difference. Often the ending of the story leaves us wanting more. Playing through *Diablo I*, making your way further, further and further into the seemingly never ending dungeon you are finally rewarded for all of your efforts by facing down your foe. The ending (SPOILER ALERT) is not a happy one and it is one that left the player wanting more. Seeing your avatar choose to take the stone containing Diablo into themselves to protect the world, and having the game end in that moment is jarring. It keeps you thinking about the story, it sticks with you.

When we think about Act 3 of tHJ for books and films this is where the hero has their time to reflect on growth. For those playing video games this is the time for the player to reflect. You get to think of all you did to arrive at the final moment, the choices you made, the journey you experienced. Further, games give us the chance to go back on that journey again and to see how different choices can lead to different endings.

Self-reflection and self-fulfillment are both integrally tied to happiness and long-term life satisfaction (Elliot & Coker, 2011; Haybron, 2008; Rosenberg, 2009; Richards, Campenni, & Muse-Burke, 2010). Although not explicitly linked in the scientific literature, it seems reasonable to hypothesize that following tHJ the player may also have developed a greater sense of self-compassion (i.e., being kind toward oneself in instance of failure), as players' abilities (and inabilities) dynamically grown and adjust to overcome in-game challenges through their journey. The development of self-compassion has been linked to positive psychological functioning and measures of happiness (Neff, Rude, & Kirkpatrick, 2007).

Lastly, undertaking tHJ in the relatively consequence free space of video games in and of itself can promote a sense of happiness and psychological well-being. Bentham (1970) defines happiness as the sum of pleasures minus pains. If this is the case, then the video games may be the ultimate learning ground for exploring different aspects of ourselves in ways that encourage happiness and long-term life satisfaction.

Concluding Thoughts

Progressing through the Hero's Journey in a role-playing game creates a create space for reflection, opportunities to question our beliefs or understanding of the world, and to analyze our behavior across a wide variety of contexts. Just as a good book or film can stick with us, so too can the story we go on in a game. We might identify with the character, feel as though their journey was our journey. Having this virtual adventure changes us and can help us change our ideas about who we are and how we operate in the world. This process is referred to as story editing (Wilson, 2011). Editing our own story is in part how we grow and change across the lifespan (e.g., telling the story of being a survivor rather than the story of being a victim).

As stated by Parker and Horton (1994), "The universe is made up of stories rather than atoms (p. 82)." In the Hero's Journey—the mono*myth*—the core belief is the ability for people of all ages can grow through adversity. The monomyth encourages us to be aware and mindful of what we have in the present, even the mundane. It tells us that we can overcome the challenges before us by starting small, learning along the way, and drawing on friends and mentors to guide us. The monomyth is upfront with the fact that life is hard and that sometimes you will fail. It also is quite blunt about how coming home after such a journey will change you, your perspective on the world, and the world's perspective of you. It is about taking a leap of faith, persisting through the challenges, and reflecting on how far you have come when you reach the end. And lastly, the Hero's Journey is a circle. Each Departure leads to Initiation leads to Return leads to Departure ad nauseum. This provides a roadmap for continuous and perpetual growth should a person heed the call.

References

Bentham, J. (1970). An introduction to the principles of morals and legislation. In J. H. Burns & H. L. A. Hart (Eds.), *Collected works of Jeremy Bentham*. London: Athlone.

Bethesda Game Studios. (2011). *The Elder Scrolls V: Skyrim* [Video game]. Bethesda Softworks.

Bioware. (2014). *Dragon Age: Inquisition* [Video game]. Electronic Arts.

Blasko, D. G., Lum, H. C., White, M. M., & Drabnik, H. B. (2014). Individual differences in the enjoyment and effectiveness of serious games. In T. Connolly, T. Hainey, E. Boyle, G. Baxter, & P. Moreno-Ger (Eds.), *Psychology, pedagogy, and assessment in serious games* (pp. 153–174). Hershey, PA: IGI Global.

Blizzard. (2004). *World of Warcraft* [Video game]. Blizzard Entertainment.

Blizzard North. (2000). *Diablo* II [Video game]. Blizzard Entertainment.

Bowman, S. L. (2010). Role-playing as an alteration of identity. In *The functions of role-playing games: How participants create community, solve problems, and explore identity*. Jefferson, NC: McFarland & Co. Inc.

Campbell, J. (2008). The Monomyth. In *The hero with a thousand faces: The collected works of Joseph Campbell* (3rd ed., 1–32). Novato, CA: New World Library.

Csikszentmihalyi, M. (1975). *Beyond boredom and anxiety*. San Francisco, CA: Josey-Bass Publishers.

Christy, K., & Fox, J. (2016). Transportability and presence as predictors of avatar identification within narrative video games. *Cyberpsychology, Behavior, and Social Networking, 19*(4), 283–287. https://doi.org/10.1089/cyber.215.0474.

Cryptic Studios. (2016). *Neverwinter* [Video game]. Perfect World Entertainment.

Darvasi, P., Farber, M., & Rivers, S. (2019). *Museum of me: Exploring identity with what remains of Edith Finch*. Presented at Games for Change. New York City.

Deci, E. L., & Ryan, R. M. (2008). Facilitating optimal motivation and psychological well-being across life's domains. *Canadian Psychology, 49*(1), 14–23.

DeSteno, D., Gross, J. J., & Kubzansky, L. (2013). Affective science and health: The importance of emotion and emotion regulation. *Health Psychology, 34*(5), 474–486. https://doi.org/10.1037/a0030259.

Deterding, S. (2018). Gamification in management: Between choice architecture and humanistic design. *Journal of Management Inquiry, 28*(2), 131–136. https://doi.org/10.1177/1056492618790912.

Ducheneaut, N., Wen, M. H., Yee, N., & Wadley, G. (2009, April). Body and mind: A study of avatar personalization in three virtual worlds. In *Proceedings of the SIGCHI conference on human factors in computing systems* (pp. 1151–1160). ACM.

Dunlap, K. (2019). Beyond empathy 101: Digging deep into empathy, ethics, and game design. Presented at the Games 4 Change Festival. New York, NY.

Dweck, C. S. (2007). The perils and promises of praise. *Educational Leadership, 65*(2), 34–39.

Elliot, I., & Coker, S. (2011). Independent self-construal, self-reflection, and self-rumination: A path model for predicting happiness. *Australian Journal of Psychology, 60*(3), 127–134.

Frasca, G. (2003). *Rethinking agency and immersion: Videogames as a means of consciousness raising*. Retrieved from http://www.siggraph.org/artdesign/gallery/S01/essays/0378.pdf.

FromSoftware. (2011). *Dark souls* [Video game]. Namco Bandai Games.

FromSoftware. (2019). *Sekiro* [Video game]. Activision.

Gabriel, S., & Young, A. (2011). Becoming a Vampire without being bitten: The narrative collective-assimilation hypothesis. *Psychological Science, 22*(8), 990–994. https://doi.org/10.1177/0956797611415541.

Gee, J. P. (2003). *What video games have to teach us about learning and literacy*. New York, NY: Palgrave.

Giant Sparrow. (2017). *What Remains of Edith Finch* [Video game]. Santa Monica, CA: Anna Purna Interactive.

Grace, L., Dunlap, K., Datu, C., & Rice, J. (2016). *Community engagement at the intersection of games and news*. Presented at the Community Management

Summit, Game Developers Conference, San Francisco, CA. https://www.gdcvault.com/browse/gdc-16/play/1023407.

Haybron, D. M. (2008). Happiness, the self and human flourishing. *Utilitas, 20*(1), 21–49.

Hodent, C. (2017). *The gamer's brain: How neuroscience and UX can impact video game design*. Boca Raton: CRC Press.

Jagoda, P., Gilliam, M., McDonald, P., & Russell, C. (2015). Worlding through play: Alternate reality games, large-scale learning, and the source. *American Journal of Play, 8*(1), 74–100. Retrieved from http://proxyau.wrlc.org/login?url=; https://search-proquest-com.proxyau.wrlc.org/docview/1729233959?accountid=8285.

Juul, J. (2013). *The art of failure*. Cambridge, MA: MIT Press.

Klimmt, C., Hefner, H., & Vorderer, P. (2009). The video game experience as "true" identification: A theory of enjoyable alterations of players' self-perception. *Communication Theory, 19*, 351–373.

Kowert, R., Griffiths, M., & Oldmeadow, J. A. (2012). Geek or Chic? Emerging stereotypes of online gamers. *Bulletin of Science, Technology & Society, 32*(6), 471–479. https://doi.org/10.1177/0270467612469078.

Lawson, G. (2005). The hero's journey as a developmental metaphor for counseling. *Journal of Humanistic Counseling, Education, and Development, 44*, 134–145. https://onlinelibrary.wiley.com/doi/abs/10.1002/j.2164-490X.2005.tb00026.x.

Lazzaro, N. (2004). *Why we play games: Four keys to more emotion without story*. XEO Design. Retrieved from https://pdfs.semanticscholar.org/2c62/e7ddb42506beb06cad57c7bd9ee4a93b714c.pdf.

McGonigal, J. (2015). *SuperBetter*. New York, NY: Penguin Books.

McGonigal, J. [TED]. (2010). *Gaming can make a better world | Jane McGonigal*. [Video File]. Retrieved from https://youtu.be/dE1DuBesGYM.

Neff, K. D., Rude, S. S., & Kirkpatrick, K. L. (2007). An examination of self-compassion in relation to positive psychological functioning and personality traits. *Journal of Research in Personality, 41*(4), 908–916.

Nintendo. (1992). *Mario kart* [Video game]. Nintendo.

Nintendo. (2017). *Legend of Zelda: Breath of the wild* [Video game]. Nintendo.

Parker, R. J., & Horton, H. S. (1994). A typology of ritual: Paradigms for healing and empowerment. *Counseling and Values, 40*, 82–97.

Pringle, H. (2015). Conjuring the ideal self: An investigation of self-presentation in video game avatars. *Press Start, 2*(1), 1–20. Retrieved from http://press-start.gla.ac.uk.

Przybylski, A. K., Weinstein, N., Murayama, K., Lynch, M. F., & Ryan, R. M. (2012). The ideal self at play: The appeal of video games that let you be all you can be. *Psychological Science, 23*(1), 69–76.

Richards, K., Campenni, C., & Muse-Burke, J. (2010). Self-care and well-being in mental health professionals: The mediating effects of self-awareness and mindfulness. *Journal of Mental Health Counseling, 32*(3), 247–264.

Rosenberg, L. R. (2009). Transforming leadership: Reflective practice and the enhancement of happiness. *Reflective Practice, 11*(1), 9–18.

Ryan, R. M., Rigby, C. S., & Przybylski, A. (2006). The motivational pull of video games: A self-determination theory approach. *Motivation and Emotion, 30*(4), 344–360. https://doi.org/10.1007/s11031-006-9051-8.

Sherry, J. (2004). Flow and media enjoyment. *Communication Theory, 14*, 328–347. https://doi.org/10.1093/ct/14.4.328.

Sutton-Smith, B. (1997). Rhetorics of self. In *The Ambiguity of Play*. Cambridge, MA: Harvard University Press.

Turkay, S., & Kinzer, C. K. (2014). The effects of avatar-based customization on player identification. *International Journal of Gaming and Computer-Mediated Simulations,* 6(1), 1–26. https://doi.org/10.4018/ijgcms.2014010101, http://gamesresearchlab.com/wp-content/uploads/2015/11/Avatar-Based-Cusomization.pdf.

Waggoner, Z. (2009). *My avatar, myself; Identity in video role-playing games.* Jefferson, NC: McFarland.

Wilson, T. (2011). *Redirect: The surprising new science of psychological change little.* New York, NY: Brown and Company.

Wrisinger, C. (2014). *"Link"ing monomyth and video games: How the Legend of Zelda connects myth to modern media* (Unpublished thesis). University of Central Missouri. https://centralspace.ucmo.edu/bitstream/handle/123456789/324/Wrisinger201420_T_Linking.pdf?sequence=8&isAllowed=y.

CHAPTER 10

Extra Lives

Raffael Boccamazzo

Abstract This chapter discusses the importance of stories in portraying factors of resilience in overcoming posttraumatic reactions that may result from the experience of potential trauma events. Video games, especially, offer the opportunity to explore our own sense of resilience through the lens of interactive fictional characters. This chapter examines posttraumatic reactions and potential trauma events as well as discusses the differences between typical posttraumatic reactions versus long-term pathology resulting from potential trauma events. Resilience and vulnerability to long-term posttraumatic effects are also discussed, highlighting various pre-event, peri-event, and post-event factors. The chapter concludes by outlining the interrelated nature of meaning-making and posttraumatic growth and how they may aid in resilience and growth.

Keywords Trauma · Posttraumatic effects · Posttraumatic stress disorder · Resilience · Vulnerability · Posttraumatic growth · Video games

---

R. Boccamazzo (✉)
Take This, Seattle, WA, USA
e-mail: doctorb@takethis.org

R. Kowert (ed.), *Video Games and Well-being*,
Palgrave Studies in Cyberpsychology,
https://doi.org/10.1007/978-3-030-32770-5_10

Hardship and strife in one's life is nothing new. Every good story involves tension and change through the process of overcoming obstacles. The book *Exploring the Psychological Benefits of Hardship* (Jayawickreme & Blackie, 2016) states the idea of suffering is a ubiquitous, essential predecessor of personal, emotional growth. It notes that Biblical accounts of suffering and triumph frame it as a divine test with a person's triumph being proof of their spiritual and personal righteousness and worth. The desire to see protagonists beat the odds and exit their suffering better than they began is woven into the fabric of our morality tales. In other words, being resilient is perceived as a good thing which imparts hope for a better future, and beyond morality tales, tension and growth just makes for good stories!

Video games are no exception to this concept of growth through triumph. Can you imagine if Bowser showed up to kidnap Princess Peach, Mario said, "Hey, man! Not cool!" and Bowser growled, "Oh, really?! You're right! I should stop trying to conquer the Mushroom Kingdom." Would people play that game? Probably not. It is boring watching, reading, or playing stories where characters do not grow or change. When there is no tension in the story, there is no emotional investment from the viewers (or players in this example). In the first-person shooter game *Destiny 2* (Bungie, 2017), a powerful enemy strips the noble Guardians of their powers, setting in motion the Guardians' fight to regain their powers and their status as protectors of a dwindling humanity. Alistair in *Dragon Age: Origins* (Bioware, 2009) and Link from the *Legend of Zelda* (Nintendo, 1986) franchise are orphans who overcome multiple obstacles set in their path. In *Final Fantasy IV* (Square, 1991) the main character Cecil must literally overcome his own dark self to find personal redemption and save the entire world.

These are not simple challenges these heroes face. In some cases, they face the threat of literally world-altering tragedy. This begs a few seemingly simple questions with some surprisingly complicated answers. How do these characters overcome significant threats to self and others with their mental health unaffected? How do they triumph when others fail? Why do some people develop significant, lasting symptoms of trauma, and why do others move on with their mental health largely unaffected? Do some people even emerge better than they were before when faced with exceptional suffering? This chapter answers these questions by examining trauma, PTSD, and factors of vulnerability and resilience through the lens of video games. Video games offer us the historically unprecedented opportunity to engage with these kinds of events from a fictional perspective at our leisure. One can begin and end when one chooses. They provide us a safe framework of fiction by which we might explore our own vulnerabilities and triumphs through the actions of interactive characters. The stories that they offer allow us to "live" through potentially world-shattering events and overcome them from the safety and comfort of our own home (often with convenient snacks). This provides an incredible opportunity to engage and immerse oneself in a range of experiences that can subtly teach us the skills and tools needed to foster resilience in the face of trauma (for more on the role of games and learning, particularly through RPGs, see Chapters 1 and 9 in this volume).

This chapter will begin by defining the differences between trauma events and routine stressors. Next, by examining the symptoms of posttraumatic stress disorder (PTSD) and some of the factors that may contribute to vulnerability and resilience. This chapter will conclude by examining the ways in which we can reestablish health and safety after suffering from PTSD.

What Is Trauma?

Certainly, we hear the term "trauma" used with some frequency in day-to-day life and in the media. However, what does it actually mean in a strict sense? Is it the same as the typical stressors and hardships that we all routinely face in the course of our lives? If it is different than routine stressors, how does trauma affect people?

Potential Trauma Events

While the definitions of trauma and posttraumatic reactions vary in the scientific literature, generally speaking the term *posttraumatic reaction* refers to the long-term, cognitive, emotional, and behavioral effects that a *potentially traumatic event* (PTE; a term coined by Shalev, 2002) might have on a person after the PTE ends. In other words, posttraumatic reactions are lingering injuries upon one's ability to cope with stressors, brought about by significant events.

Broadly defined, a PTE is an inescapable event that is stressful enough to completely overwhelm a person's ability to cope (van der Kolk & Fisler, 1995). The fifth edition of *Diagnostic and Statistical Manual of Mental Disorders* (DSM-5) diagnostic criteria for PTSD more narrowly defines

PTEs as exposure to actual death, threats of death, serious injury, or sexual violence (American Psychiatric Association [APA], 2013). It also goes further and defines the types of events which qualify as exposure to the dangers above: events where the person is the one directly in danger and survives; event involving those who witness danger affecting others; and events involving people who learn about the accidental or violent death of a loved one. Taking these one at a time, let's figure out what real-world events might qualify as PTEs, according to the DSM-5.

The first PTE type involves events where a person is the one in serious danger and survives the encounter. This might include a gravely wounded combat veteran or a person who survives rape. No reasonable person would say those are safe situations, and obviously both examples involve a person who reasonably fears for their safety and/or their own life.

The second PTE type includes those who witness a PTE affecting other people. This could include events like witnessing a loved one grievously injured in a car accident or watching paramedics resuscitate a friend. Of note, this criterion also includes those whose actions were responsible for the danger or injury to others such as a person who causes a car accident or even the perpetrators of criminal acts. It also includes emergency responders like firefighters and police officers who routinely and repetitively witness the results of harm to others.

Finally, the third PTE type includes those who learn about the accidental or violent death (or threatened death) of a loved one. An example of this would be families of emergency responders or military personnel who learn about the deaths of their family members.

It's important to note that the specific examples above do not represent an exhaustive list of the types of events that could qualify as PTEs. The more important factor is the degree to which they expose a person to perceived or actual danger in some manner, as well as the manner in which these factors overwhelm a person's ability to cope with the danger.

Cecil the Dark Knight and Rydia

In the context of this above criteria of a PTE (i.e., exposure to self or others in grave danger), let's examine the now-classic video game *Final Fantasy IV*—marketed as *Final Fantasy II* upon its original release in the United States (Square, 1991). *Final Fantasy IV* presents many characters who face overwhelming events, but there are two characters, in particular, who stand out: Cecil the Dark Knight and the powerful magic user Rydia of Mist.

At the game's beginning, Cecil is the commander of a branch of his king's military. He is a loyal subject and long-time military commander who attacks a neighboring kingdom on orders from his king, convinced that they possess technology which threatens the citizens of his home kingdom. Cecil later realizes that, in following his king's orders, he murders innocent civilians in the neighboring kingdom. Despite his years of military training and experience, this event is one of several which haunt him throughout the game.

The king strips Cecil of his military command after Cecil expresses doubts about the mission. The king orders Cecil to deliver a ring to the city of Mist, which requires Cecil and his traveling companion to defeat the dragon which guards Mist. Once in Mist, the ring Cecil carries opens and releases incendiary magic, immolating the village. In the rapidly spreading inferno, Cecil and his companion notice a child crying over the lifeless body of her dead mother. In a moment of epiphany, the duo realize that the mother is a powerful magic user who summoned the guardian Mist Dragon they defeated to reach the town. Magic links creatures summoned and their summoners, and by killing the Mist Dragon, they killed the woman.

With Mist rapidly burning, Cecil and his traveling companion decide to save the young child, named Rydia. Before they can, Rydia realizes that the duo killed the Mist Dragon and subsequently her mother. Rydia, in her terror, sorrow, and rage, attacks them with her own summoned creature—a creature powerful enough to cause an earthquake which collapses the mountain pass and isolates the town from the outside world. The earthquake separates Cecil and his companion and renders Rydia unconscious. Cecil does not shirk from his pledge to rescue Rydia and carries her to the nearest safe town. Rydia does not respond to Cecil's reassurances or apologies for unknowingly killing her mother, at least until Cecil protects her from members of his former military organization who try to kill her. Cecil repeats his pledge to protect her, and she begins to slowly trust him.

How do these events meet criteria for PTEs? Cecil witnessed the deaths of others due to his own actions killing others. Rydia witnessed her family and home incinerated by Cecil and witnessed the death of her mother when Cecil and his companion slayed the mother's summoned Mist Dragon. Both Cecil and Rydia face experiences where others are both threatened and killed. Additionally, Rydia also fought back against Cecil and his companion because she perceived her own life to be in danger. These both clearly meet two criteria for types of PTEs, as defined by the DSM-5 (APA, 2013).

Typical Reactions to PTEs Versus Pathology

So far, we've discussed what PTEs are, and we even have a few concrete example, We also discussed a broad definition of posttraumatic reactions as lingering emotional, behavioral, and physical effects which may result from exposure to a PTE. That said, what are the typical reactions to PTEs, and what is the difference between that and diagnoses like PTSD?

Typical Reactions

The majority of those exposed to a PTE do not suffer long-term dysfunction but instead face a process of coping with transient stress from the extremity of the event or events (Brown & Goodman, 2005; McDonald et al., 2016; Miron, Orcutt, & Kumpula, 2014). This bears repeating. Most people exposed to a PTE do not suffer long-term dysfunction. This is the reason Shalev (2002) argued for the use of the term *potential* trauma event. Even though we know most people recover from these extreme events, what types of reactions can we expect to see from people exposed to the types of situations listed above?

The reality is that people's reactions during and after PTEs and span a wide gamut of human emotional, cognitive, and behavioral experiences. Those faced with fearful and dangerous situations often act with...well, fear. This includes all the "fight or flight" physiological reactions one might expect (e.g., racing heart, rapid breathing, sweating), but also can go so far as to include flattening of emotions ("numbness"), as well as cognitive responses such as confusion, an inability to respond to stimuli, disorientation, and dissociation (Shalev, 2002; World Health Organization, 2016). Forms of dissociation (e.g., derealization and depersonalization) are some of the more extreme reactions to PTEs, though they are not the only potential cognitive or memory disruptions that may occur. Memory disruptions may also include partial or total amnesia for the PTE, or they may only be remembered as vague sensations such as pressure on the body or smells (van der Kolk & Fisler, 1995).

Something to bear in mind: many of these reactions are adaptive. Fear, after all, is a logical and reasonable response to a realistic threat. It mobilizes the physiological responses needed to either fight or flee a threatening situation. Once the threat ends, the fear responses ideally subside, and a person returns to baseline. In some cases, this may take days or weeks, but (again) the majority of people exposed to PTEs return to normal functioning and reconstruct the narrative of their PTE in a way that allows them to move forward with their lives (Meichenbaum, 2014). Shalev (2002) described the recovery process as a transition from survival/safety-based processes to begin to internalize the extreme events of the PTEs. This logically begs the question, "What about those whose fear responses don't completely abate after the PTE ends?" That's when we start to consider various diagnoses like PTSD.

What Is PTSD?

Posttraumatic stress disorder (PTSD) is arguably the most widely recognized trauma disorder, though it's not the only one. We see trauma disorders represented in various forms (and quality of portrayal) throughout a variety of media contexts, including video games. Unfortunately, video game portrayals of trauma-related disorders are often no more than a device to motivate the character to action, instead of nuanced portrayals of actual disorders like PTSD (Eurogamer, 2015). In *American McGee's Alice* (Rogue Entertainment, 2000), we find Lewis Carroll's original characters twisted into a Victorian horror story. Alice, confined to an asylum, suffers from catatonic "madness" and a loss of reality in response to witnessing her parents die in a fire. A more compassionate portrayal is found in *Stardew Valley* (ConcernedApe, 2016), when the player meets a nonplayer character named Kent who returned from military service easily startled, frequently angry, and expressing difficulty sleeping. Through compassionate interactions with Kent, the player helps Kent address some of these concerns to live a more fulfilling life with his family.

Like all mental health diagnoses, PTSD requires a series of symptoms that significantly impair a person's functions and/or cause significant distress over a period of time. Based on the current, US diagnostic criteria (APA, 2013), there are five major components of PTSD: a person experiences a PTE, as defined above; re-experiences the PTE in various ways (e.g., intrusive memories, dissociative flashbacks, distressing dreams, or distressing reactions to reminders of the PTE); engages in persistent attempts to avoid reminders of the PTE; experiences altered cognitions (e.g., irrational guilt or beliefs about self or others) and negative moods (e.g., loss of interest in enjoyable activities, persistent fear, alienation from others, or an inability to experience positive emotions) related to the PTE; and experiences altered reactivity to stimuli (e.g., difficulties concentrating, increased startle response, irritability and anger, difficulty sleeping, or hypervigilance).

Per this diagnostic criteria, most of these domains must begin or worsen after exposure to one or more PTEs, the symptoms must last longer than 1 month, and these symptoms cannot be the result of the physiological effects of a medical condition or substance.

While it is not clear if Rydia suffers from PTSD in *Final Fantasy IV* (Square, 1991), she does display several symptoms in one scene. The heroes must travel through a mountain pass. They find their path blocked by a wall of ice, and the only member of their party with the ability to use fire magic to melt the ice is Rydia. The problem is that fire terrifies Rydia. Fire razed her village immediately after her mother died in front of her. She is initially unable or unwilling to utilize her own abilities because they remind her of the destruction of her village and the death of her mother, and she appears initially flooded with negative emotions, reacting with an angry outburst at the mention of her using fire magic. While she quickly overcomes this with the help of her friends, her reactivity to the reminders of her PTE and her avoidance of those reminders are some of the classic symptoms of PTSD if they continued to impair her functioning long-term.

Resilience and Vulnerability

By definition, PTSD is a disrupting and sometimes debilitating diagnosis, but what are the factors which contribute to people struggling with it? Additionally, we can think about resilience as a person's ability to overcome significant stressors (Meichenbaum, 2014), but what are the factors which contribute to resilience? Broadly, we can divide them into three categories: the factors from before the PTE occurs (pre-event factors), the factors at work during and immediately after the PTE (peri-event factors), and the factors which occur after the PTE ends (post-event factors).

One of the challenges in examining universal factors contributing to resilience is the variability of the people involved, trauma types, and even the definitions of trauma in the studies themselves. For example, would we expect children to be differently affected than adults? Do natural disasters affect people differently than motor vehicle accidents or military combat? How does culture play a part in posttraumatic effects? Do we see differences across genders? Given the changes in diagnostic criteria of PTSD over the years (e.g., APA, 2000, 2013), do previous studies still apply?

A meta-analysis of 77 trauma studies examined fourteen risk factors of PTSD, and suggested that drawing ubiquitous conclusions is challenging for all the reasons above, but there are some factors in resilience which can be more universally applied: pre-event psychiatric variables; peri-event factors such as the severity of the PTE; and post-event factors such as social support (Brewin, Andrews, & Valentine, 2000). They noted that peri-event and post-event factors appeared to have a greater relationship with the development of PTSD than pre-event factors, which we eventually see in the above example of the heroes needing Rydia to cast fire magic to help through the mountain pass. She eventually overcomes her fear to cast fire magic and helps the party, largely due to the post-event social support she receives, as well as a meaning shift in her personal narrative of herself as a victim of fire to an empowered wielder of fire magic who saves lives.

Pre-event Factors

In terms of the pre-event factors which contribute to resilience versus pathology, this chapter largely focuses on psychiatric variables. The nuances of demographic variables such as age, gender identity, socioeconomic status, and culture are varied and worthy of more attention than this chapter can give (e.g., Brewin et al., 2000; Howell, 2011; McDonald et al., 2016). That said, there are some biopsychosocial factors such pre-existing vulnerability to anxiety (Lin et al., 2015) may contribute to the development of PTSD when exposed to PTEs. Early family instability and a previous trauma history were also associated with vulnerability to PTSD when exposed to PTEs (Cougle, Resnick, & Kilpatrick, 2009; King, King, Foy, Keane, & Fairbank, 1999).

Certain pre-event cognitive beliefs and coping style were also associated with differing degrees of both vulnerability and resilience to PTEs. Numerous studies describe a flexible belief in one's ability to cope and a sense of optimism as protective against trauma-related pathology (Acquaye, 2017; Deković, Koning, Stams, & Buist, 2008; King et al., 1999). Essentially, a flexible, realistic, self-committed belief of, "I can do it!" appears protective. The word "flexible" should be emphasized, as there is some support for the idea that rigid beliefs in the need to be self-reliant may contribute to future vulnerability (Nanney, Wamser-Nanney, Link, Constans, & Pyne, 2018). Incidentally, one study found that cognitive flexibility after a PTE was associated with more positive outcomes, though they could not determine if that was due to pre-existing flexibility (Ben-Zion et al., 2018). Perhaps unsurprisingly, beliefs of one's inability to handle adversity may contribute to a feedback loop of avoidance behaviors (Hashoul-Andary et al., 2016).

Avoidant coping styles, versus active management of emotional and behavioral symptoms were associated with more substantial long-term trauma-related problems (Iacoviello & Charney, 2014; Pooley, Cohen, O'Conner, & Taylor, 2013).

We do not know much about the backgrounds and childhoods of most of the characters of *Final Fantasy IV* (Square, 1991), but given Cecil's age and military training, it seems likely that he possesses a certain resolute, optimistic attitude about his own abilities to cope with stress that may be contributing factors as to why we do not see many overt symptoms of PTSD after the deaths of civilians in the neighboring kingdom and destruction of Mist. He quickly decides on a plan to address them and moves ahead with them, confronting his discomfort. Meanwhile, Rydia's young age seems to leave her more vulnerable to later pathological symptoms, as we do eventually see.

Peri-Event Factors

Certain peri-event factors, in particular, stand out as potential contributors to people's vulnerability and resilience to PTEs. The first is the nature of the PTEs, namely the severity, duration, and a person's emotional and physical proximity to the event. People who are more closely emotionally invested in the event (e.g., losing a parent in a violent accident), as well as those who are physically closer to the event may increase the risk of long-term pathology (Hughes et al., 2011; Miron et al., 2014). As a seemingly opposite corollary to some of the above pre-event cognitive factors, it has been suggested that perceptions of helplessness, powerlessness, and the inability to escape the PTE may contribute to future development of posttraumatic symptoms (Foa, Zinbarg, & Rothbaum, 1992).

Above, we discussed a variety of reactions that a person may display in response to PTEs. Of those, one of the most concerning for future functioning is dissociation. Dissociative experiences predicted greater likelihood of posttraumatic symptoms (Miron et al., 2014), and people vulnerable to dissociation as a coping skill during the event are prone to keep doing so once the event subsides (van der Kolk & Fisler, 1995).

Returning to our in-game examples, Rydia may be more vulnerable to long-term pathology due to both her emotional and physical proximity to danger and loss during her PTEs. She watched a primary caregiver suddenly die in front of her. In terms of childhood interpersonal connectedness, the parent/child relationship is ideally the closest emotional relationship there is. Immediately afterwards, her home burns around her, leaving her physically trapped between the massive blaze immolating her entire community and the person who killed her mother.

Post-event Factors

The Legend of Zelda (Nintendo, 1986) tells us, “It’s dangerous to go alone.” Trauma research substantiates this notion, as social support stands out as a powerful protective factor against future dysfunction in the aftermath of a PTE. In fact, Brewing et al. (2000) found that a lack of it to be the strongest predictor of posttraumatic symptoms after a PTE. Social support may be related to perceptions of agency and the ability to mobilize help and safety resources when needed (Deković et al., 2008).

Meaning-making and *posttraumatic growth* (Tedeschi & Calhoun, 1996) both bear special mention, especially as they are interrelated. The ability to derive meaning from events is an integral part of many therapeutic modalities and approaches (e.g., Beck, 1995; Frankl, 1959; Kopp, 1972) and is important for fostering resilience and recovery from PTEs. Meaning helps us, “…interpret the past, negotiate the present, and anticipate [the] future.” (Meichenbaum, 2014, p. 331) We create meaning in our lives to interpret the events that occur, and some trauma theorists view PTEs as a sort of “plot twist” in our life narratives that shatters one’s assumptions in one’s place in the world and how it works (Jirek, 2017). This can result in trauma survivors transposing their trauma meanings onto seemingly innocuous events and occurrences, instead of deriving meaning from the mundane events (van der Kolk, 2014).

Posttraumatic growth (Tedeschi & Calhoun, 2004) is a relatively recent concept; however, the idea of constructing meaning from traumatic events is an integral component. Posttraumatic growth reflects perceived positive changes in several areas of life following a PTE. Tedeschi and Calhoun’s model (2004) incorporates many of the concepts of resilience above, such as the importance of social support and the transition away from involuntary ruminations to more deliberate thought about the PTE to create positive change in a person’s world view and personal narrative, resulting in positive changes in five domains: increased appreciation of life, positive changes in interpersonal relationships, increased sense of personal strength, positively changed priorities, and a richer existential life.[1]

Helping PTE survivors take their tribulations and develop new, personal, beneficial beliefs about their self and their place in the world is a component of several approaches to recovery (e.g., Meichenbaum, 2014; Schwartz, 2016; Tadeschi & Calhoun, 2004; Williams & Poijula, 2016). Spirituality can be a component of that, as well. Depending on how religion and/or spirituality are applied, commitment to or the rejection of religion and spirituality may aid in recovery (Brown, 2009). For example, children who lost family in the September 11th terrorist attacks showed increased resilience through religious engagement (Brown & Goodman, 2005). The authors hypothesized that this was allowed the bereaved to draw ongoing feelings of connection to the family member who died, establish social connectedness with community, and create meaning from their family member's death. Interestingly, one qualitative study (Jirek, 2017) posited that social acceptability of a given trauma narrative may also be a hindrance to developing a healing narrative. In other words, if a PTE survivor does not believe that people will accept their new narrative, they hesitate to embrace it.

A poignant example of meaning, connectedness, and resilience is found in the final battle of *Final Fantasy IV* (Square, 1991). Zeromus, the final boss, nearly annihilates the assembled heroes in one blast of magic, leaving only the (now paladin) Cecil conscious. The heroes' collective allies all over the world, united in support and prayer, inspire Cecil to rise, and the spirits of lost friends appear to the heroes and inspire them to follow Cecil and defeat Zeromus. While this is not a particularly subtle example, the heroes' ability to literally rise from potential defeat was fueled directly by their willingness to draw ongoing support from those in their community, as well as the sense of connectedness and memories of those they lost along their journey to literally save the world, and one does not find much of a nobler narrative than that.

[1] It bears noting that much of the posttraumatic growth research is based on retrospective self-reports from those who survived PTEs (Jayawickreme & Blackie, 2014). In other words, people answer the question, "Do you think you're doing better than before?" Jayawickreme & Blackie (2016) suggest that ongoing research is needed to further solidify our understanding of whether or not people's positive self-perceptions conform with the perceptions of others or even against a baseline measure of something like interpersonal relationships prior to the PTE.

Putting It All Together

The scene of Rydia needing to cast fire magic in the mountain pass is an example of multiple post-event factors at work. Rydia initially refuses attempting fire magic, and turns away from the ice wall, overwhelmed with emotions. Acknowledging Rydia's fear and hesitation, as well as the reasons behind them, the party nonjudgmentally reminds her of her own agency in confronting her fears and the bravery involved in choosing to do so. They inform her that by doing this, Rydia will save lives, as danger threatens the people of Fabul (their destination city). After her friends' collective support and encouragement, Rydia finds her inner strength and casts a fire spell, clearing the way for the heroes to continue with their journey and save the world.

While this is a short cut scene, there are several factors at work that illustrate the complex nature of resilience and vulnerability. Rydia initially lost her previous social supports (her biological family and community), which was replaced by her adventuring party, but complicated by the fact that she initially perceived Cecil as responsible for her losses.

The narrative of her PTE quickly changed, first in discovering that Cecil was unknowingly tricked into killing her mother and burning her village, and then quickly finding herself protected by Cecil and others. She found safety and support in her new companions. Rydia's companions later help her confront her fears of fire and construct a new narrative, namely that Rydia is a hero for facing her fears and helping to literally save lives. Throughout the remainder of the game, she increasingly devotes her actions to others, nearly sacrificing herself to protect her friends.

Cecil's arc is a bit different in that he did not appear to suffer the same degree of effects from his PTEs as Rydia. Firstly, Cecil's personal narrative remains fairly consistent: he views himself as a soldier tricked into betraying his values of trying to do the right thing in how he acts. It could be argued that he perceives himself as a victim of someone else's deception. Cecil also never loses his support system the same way that Rydia does; he retains his best friend Kain and his love interest Rosa. Cecil certainly ruminates on the PTEs and expresses tremendous guilt, but he does not appear to display any avoidant symptoms. In fact, Cecil actively seeks redemption by confronting his own dark side (metaphorically and literally) anthropomorphized as a mirror image of himself. Cecil refrains from fighting this dark side, accepting it as an inescapable part of himself and his journey toward betterment instead, and emerges from the confrontation as a paladin, an embodiment of goodness and justice. Like Rydia, Cecil seeks narrative change, namely in the form of redemption and becomes a protector of others. This growth allows him to not only find a measure of peace with his PTEs, but engage in posttraumatic growth and become the hero, friend, and husband he always wanted to be.

Conclusion

Posttraumatic effects are the behavioral, emotional, and cognitive injuries to the self caused by potential trauma events—events which are often beyond our control and push our coping skills to the limits. There are a number of factors (e.g., social support, active symptom management, flexible, optimistic expectations of ourselves) which can protect us from lingering emotional symptoms in many cases. Even if people find themselves affected by long-term posttraumatic effects from PTEs, there is hope for a renewed meaning and triumph, much like many of our favorite characters.

We have no shortage of characters who grow through the process of overcoming horrifying odds and perilous dangers. Certainly, many of the examples in this chapter exemplify recovery and growth. In real life, there is no straight line to a better future like there is in many video games. There is no one code or magic spell for recovery from trauma. Still, perhaps it is helpful to think of stories as a distillation of the factors above and something we can all aspire to tapping into the strength which we have inside us to find forward momentum and growth, even in the face of sometimes overwhelming odds, changing our pain and struggles into personal triumphs.

References

Acquaye, H. E. (2017). PTSD, optimism, religious commitment, and growth as post-trauma trajectories: A structural equation modeling of former refugees. *The Professional Counselor, 7*(4), 330–348. https://doi.org/10.15241/hea.7.4.330.

American Psychiatric Association. (2000). *Diagnostic and statistical manual of mental disorders* (4th ed., Text Revision). Washington, DC: Author.

American Psychiatric Association. (2013). *Diagnostic and statistical manual of mental disorders* (5th ed.). Washington, DC: Author.

American Psychological Association. (n.d.). *Trauma*. Retrieved May 29, 2019, from https://www.apa.org/topics/trauma.

Beck, J. S. (1995). *Cognitive therapy: Basics and beyond*. New York: Guilford Press.

Ben-Zion, Z., Fine, N. B., Keynan, N. J., Admon, R., Green, N., Halevi, M., … Shalev, A. Y. (2018). Cognitive Flexibility predicts PTSD symptoms: Observational and interventional studies. *Frontiers in Psychiatry, 9*. https://doi.org/10.3389/fpsyt.2018.00477.

Bioware. (2009). *Dragon age: Origins* [Computer software]. Redwood City, CA: Electronic Arts, Inc.

Brewin, C. R., Andrews, B., & Valentine, J. D. (2000). Meta-analysis of risk factors for posttraumatic stress disorder in trauma-exposed adults. *Journal of Consulting and Clinical Psychology, 68*(5), 748–766. https://doi.org/10.1037/0022-006x.68.5.748.

Brown, L. S. (2009). *Cultural competence in trauma therapy: Beyond the flashback*. Washington, DC: American Psychological Association.

Brown, E. J., & Goodman, R. F. (2005). Childhood traumatic grief: An exploration of the construct in children bereaved on September 11. *Journal of Clinical Child and Adolescent Psychology, 34*(2), 248–259. https://doi.org/10.1037/e416482005-035.

Bungie. (2017). *Destiny 2* [Computer software]. Santa Monica, CA: Activision, Inc.

ConcernedApe. (2016). *Stardew Valley* [Computer software]. London: Chucklefish Games.

Cougle, J. R., Resnick, H., & Kilpatrick, D. G. (2009). A prospective examination of PTSD symptoms as risk factors for subsequent exposure to potentially traumatic events among women. *Journal of Abnormal Psychology, 118*, 405–411. https://doi.org/10.1037/a0015370.

Deković, M., Koning, I. M., Stams, G. J., & Buist, K. L. (2008). Factors associated with traumatic symptoms and internalizing problems among adolescents who experienced a traumatic event. *Anxiety Stress and Coping, 21*(4), 377–386. https://doi.org/10.1080/10615800701791161.

Eurogamer. (2015, October 28). *PTSD in video games—Low batteries*. Retrieved May 26, 2019, from https://www.youtube.com/watch?v=2Fs3BBynQgE.

Foa, E. B., Zinbarg, R., & Rothbaum, B. O. (1992). Uncontrollability and unpredictability in post-traumatic stress disorder: An animal model. *Psychological Bulletin, 112*(2), 218–238. https://doi.org/10.1037/0033-2909.112.2.218.

Frankl, V. (1959). *Man's search for meaning*. Boston: Beacon Press.

Hashoul-Andary, R., Assayag-Nitzan, Y., Yuval, K., Aderka, I. M., Litz, B., & Bernstein, A. (2016). A longitudinal study of emotional distress intolerance and psychopathology following exposure to a potentially traumatic event in a community sample. *Cognitive Therapy and Research, 40*(1), 1–13. https://doi.org/10.1007/s10608-015-9730-4.

Howell, K. H. (2011). Resilience and psychopathology in children exposed to family violence. *Aggression and Violent Behavior, 16*(6), 562–569. https://doi.org/10.1016/j.avb.2011.09.001.

Hughes, M., Brymer, M., Chiu, W. T., Fairbank, J. A., Jones, R. T., Pynoos, R. S., … Kessler, R. C. (2011). Posttraumatic stress among students after the shootings at Virginia Tech. *Psychological Trauma: Theory, Research, Practice, and Policy, 3*(4), 403–411. https://doi.org/10.1037/a0024565.

Iacoviello, B. M., & Charney, D. S. (2014). Psychosocial facets of resilience: Implications for preventing posttrauma psychopathology, treating trauma survivors, and enhancing community resilience. *European Journal of Psychotraumatology, 5*(1), 23970. https://doi.org/10.3402/ejpt.v5.23970.

Jayawickreme, E., & Blackie, L. E. (2014). Post-traumatic growth as positive personality change: Evidence, controversies and future directions. *European Journal of Personality, 28*(4), 312–331. https://doi.org/10.1002/per.1963.

Jayawickreme, E., & Blackie, L. E. (2016). *Exploring the psychological benefits of hardship: A critical reassessment of posttraumatic growth.* New York: Springer.

Jirek, S. L. (2017). Narrative reconstruction and post-traumatic growth among trauma survivors: The importance of narrative in social work research and practice. *Qualitative Social Work: Research and Practice, 16*(2), 166–188. https://doi.org/10.1177/1473325016656046.

King, D. W., King, L. A., Foy, D. W., Keane, T. M., & Fairbank, J. A. (1999). Posttraumatic stress disorder in a national sample of female and male Vietnam veterans: Risk factors, war-zone stressors, and resilience-recovery variables. *Journal of Abnormal Psychology, 108*(1), 164–170. https://doi.org/10.1037//0021-843x.108.1.164.

Kopp, S. B. (1972). *If you meet the Buddha on the road, kill him! The pilgrimage of psychotherapy patients.* Palo Alto, CA: Science and Behavior Books Inc.

Lin, T., Vaisvaser, S., Fruchter, E., Admon, R., Wald, I., Pine, D. S., … Hendler, T. (2015). A neurobehavioral account for individual differences in resilience to chronic military stress. *Psychological Medicine, 45*(5), 1011–1023. https://doi.org/10.1017/s0033291714002013.

Mcdonald, S. E., Shin, S., Corona, R., Maternick, A., Graham-Bermann, S. A., Ascione, F. R., & Williams, J. H. (2016). Children exposed to intimate partner violence: Identifying differential effects of family environment on children's trauma and psychopathology symptoms through regression mixture models. *Child Abuse & Neglect, 58*, 1–11. https://doi.org/10.1016/j.chiabu.2016.06.010.

Meichenbaum, D. (2014). Ways to bolster resilience in traumatized clients: Implications for psychotherapists. *Journal of Constructivist Psychology, 27*(4), 329–336. https://doi.org/10.1080/10720537.2013.833064.

Miron, L. R., Orcutt, H. K., & Kumpula, M. J. (2014). Differential predictors of transient stress versus posttraumatic stress disorder: Evaluating risk following targeted mass violence. *Behavior Therapy, 45*(6), 791–805. https://doi.org/10.1016/j.beth.2014.07.005.

Nanney, J. T., Wamser-Nanney, R. A., Linke, L. H., Constans, J. I., & Pyne, J. M. (2018). Pretrauma power and control beliefs and posttraumatic stress: A longitudinal study of combat soldiers. *Journal of Traumatic Stress, 31*(3), 427–436. https://doi.org/10.1002/jts.22294.

Nintendo. (1986). *The Legend of Zelda* [Nintendo entertainment system software]. Kyoto, Japan: Nintendo.

Pooley, J. A., Cohen, L., O'Connor, M., & Taylor, M. (2013). Posttraumatic stress and posttraumatic growth and their relationship to coping and self-efficacy in Northwest Australian cyclone communities. *Psychological Trauma: Theory, Research, Practice, and Policy, 5*(4), 392–399. https://doi.org/10.1037/a0028046.

Rogue Entertainment. (2000). *American McGee's Alice* [Computer software]. Redwood City, CA: Electronic Arts, Inc.

Schwartz, A. (2016). *The complex PTSD workbook: A mind-body approach to regaining emotional control & becoming whole*. Berkeley, CA: Althea Press.

Shalev, A. Y. (2002). Acute stress reactions in adults. *Biological Psychiatry, 51*(7), 532–543. https://doi.org/10.1016/s0006-3223(02)01335-5.

Square. (1991). *Final Fantasy IV* [Super Nintendo entertainment system software]. Tokyo, Japan: Square.

Tedeschi, R. G., & Calhoun, L. G. (1996). The posttraumatic growth inventory: Measuring the positive legacy of trauma. *Journal of Traumatic Stress, 9*(3), 455–471. https://doi.org/10.1007/BF02103658.

Tedeschi, R. G., & Calhoun, L. G. (2004). Target article: Posttraumatic growth: Conceptual foundations and empirical evidence. *Psychological Inquiry, 15*, 1–18. https://doi.org/10.1207/s15327965pli1501_01.

van der Kolk, B. A. (2014). *The body keeps the score: Brain, mind, and body in the healing of trauma*. New York: Penguin Books.

van der Kolk, B. A., & Fisler, R. (1995). Dissociation and the fragmentary nature of traumatic memories: Overview and exploratory study. *Journal of Traumatic Stress, 8*(4), 505–525. https://doi.org/10.1002/jts.2490080402.

Williams, M. B., & Poijula, S. (2016). *The PTSD workbook: Simple, effective techniques for overcoming traumatic stress symptoms*. Oakland, CA: New Harbinger Publications.

World Health Organization. (2016). *International statistical classification of diseases and related health problems* (10th revision). Retrieved June 29, 2019, from https://icd.who.int/browse10/2016/en.

CHAPTER 11

Concluding Comments

Rachel Kowert

Abstract This chapter provides an overview of the content contained within the volume and provides suggestions for future research.

Keywords Video games · Well-being · Growth

Saving princesses. Slaying dragons. Going on wild adventures with a band of misfits. Digital games have been providing us with entertainment for decades and have become a centerpiece of modern society. No longer confined to dedicated gaming consoles, video games are now available to be played on our computers, phones, and smart watches. Despite their popularity, they have garnered a negative reputation as frivolous activities that are waste of time at best and vehicles for violence, aggression, and social dysfunction at their worst (Kowert, Festl, & Quandt, 2014; Kowert, Griffiths, & Oldmeadow, 2012). As video games have come to be ubiquitous with modern life there remains something notably missing from their public discourse: their potential to positively impact our psychological well-being.

R. Kowert (✉)
Take This, Seattle, WA, USA

R. Kowert (ed.), *Video Games and Well-being*,
Palgrave Studies in Cyberpsychology,
https://doi.org/10.1007/978-3-030-32770-5_11

No longer a childhood pastime, video games are an integral part of our lives and mirrors of society and ourselves. Unbeknownst to many, while gamers have been exploring the vast lands of *Hyrule*, defeating dragons in *Azeroth*, and searching for Princess Peach, they have also been learning, practicing, and refining a wide variety of skills to foster happier and more satisfied lives. The essays within this collection drew from research in psychology, education, ludology, media studies, and communication science to demonstrate how video game mechanics and narratives teach players a range of skills associated with increased psychological well-being, including flexible thinking, openness to experience, self-care, a growth mindset, solution-focused thinking, persistence, self-discovery, and resilience.

Chapter 1 set the groundwork for exploring how video games are similar to other forms of media we have long enjoyed for leisure and skill building, such as reading a book or learning to play a new instrument. While video games are often thought of as a separate (potentially destructive) category of entertainment, in the end all forms of media are more similar than dissimilar. This chapter elaborated on the mechanisms that underlie video games' capability to foster learning and growth, including their ability to induce a state of flow (Csikszentmihalyi, 1975, 1991). Flow states are key to video games' functionality as a learning tool, as research has found them to be a strong predictor for learning and knowledge transfer (Webster, Trevino, & Ryan, 1993), particularly in relation to video games and virtual worlds (Choi & Baek, 2011; Hamari et al., 2016; Rossin, Ro, Klein, & Guo, 2009; for more see Kiili, 2005).

Once the tools underlying video games' capacity to impact psychological growth were outlined, the essays in this volume dove deeper into how and why the unique characteristics of video games influence our thoughts and behaviors in ways that can positively influence our well-being. This began with an exploration of one of the most valuable tools in a gamers' toolbox—the reset button. Lucky for us, the opportunity to reset and start again is not only available for our 100th run of the Cave of Wonders in the NES classic *Disney's Aladdin* (Virgin Interactive, 1993). In our out-of-game lives, "resets" occur with mindfulness, patience, and the evolution of our personalities. While our personality is often thought of as an immutable feature of who we are, rigidly dictating our thoughts and actions, Chapter 2 revealed quite the opposite. Our personality is malleable over time and knowing this is key to long-lasting and meaningful change. Another important tool among gamers are guides and maps. Chapter 3 explored the role that mental maps play in our daily lives through the lens of affect theory and the practice of face-work. By understanding the tools needed to create such a map to explore and analyze the world around us, we are better able to ascribe meaning and draw insight into our everyday experiences and challenges (both positive and negative).

Chapters 4 through 8 examined how some of the more technical attributes of video games are also mechanisms for change. Chapter 4 examined how the avatars that we choose to navigate the tools of gaming worlds can influence the way we see ourselves both in- and out-of-game, whereas Chapter 5 examined how feedback loops often used video game design provide the foundation for a growth mindset. Building on this, Chapter 6 addressed how skill profiles of in-game characters can provide insight into solution-finding approaches to better understand our in- and out-of-game strengths, including resilience.

The final chapters in the volume returned to exploring specific facets of well-being that are modeled and explored through video game mechanics and content. This began in Chapter 7 with a discussion of mindfulness, which has been linked to various facets of well-being (Brown & Ryan, 2003). While the fast-paced nature of video games may seem to be the antithesis of the fast-paced nature of video games, Chapter 8 discussed how flow within video games provide the opportunity to increase awareness toward our inner and outer experiences even in fast-paced environments (Sliwinski, Katsikitis, & Jones, 2015) and how overcoming difficult in-game challenges that are created through the structure of the game, such as defeating a Lynel in Breath of the Wild (Nintendo, 2018), can lead to positive psychological growth and motivation to pursue and overcome even more difficult challenges.

Persistence was the focus of Chapters 9 and 10, the former in relation to the game mechanics and the latter in relation to game narratives. Persistence can be generally thought of as continuing on a course of action despite opposition, difficulty, or previous failures. People who are persistent often have an internal locus of control, which is the belief that individuals are responsible for their own success (Mischel, Zeiss, & Zeiss, 1974). Research has found this to be a key correlate with life-satisfaction and happiness across the lifespan (Hickson, Housley, & Boyle, 1988; Huebner, 1991; Huebner, Ash, & Laughlin, 2001; Palmore & Luikart, 1972), which are core components of our well-being. Chapter 9 delved deeper into how the narratives of the stories themselves can foster persistence through the Hero's Journey. Through role-playing this journey, players are provided the opportunity to try, fail, and try again free from the traditional repercussions associated with failure in the "real-world."

The book concluded with a discussion of how video games can provide insight into some of the more serious experiences related to well-being, post-traumatic growth following a post-traumatic experience. As discussed in Chapter 10, video games provide the unique opportunity to experience fictional versions of the darker sides of life. That is, they are able to provide a safe framework to explore our own vulnerabilities by "living through" and overcoming potentially world-shattering events from a safe and comfortable (physical and psychological) distance.

Video games are incredible tools for the unintentional learning and transfer of knowledge. While research has found video game play to promote a variety of skills and abilities, including creative thinking, problem solving, time management, and leadership skills (Bowman, Kowert, & Ferguson, 2015; Olson, 2015), researchers in the field have been calling for a greater recognition of video games as powerful tools for our well-being. That was the motivation behind the construction of this volume. Taken together, the essays collected in this volume aimed to illustrate the ways in which video games tap into our strengths and transform in-game struggles and battles into out-of-game resilience, psychological growth, and improved well-being.

It is worth noting that during the writing of this collection, new research emerged indicating that engaging in the virtual worlds of video games have the potential to dampen the expression of a stress-induced gene profile, suggesting that video game play (among what the researchers defined as "engaged" gamers) can increase one's biological defenses toward stress reactions when facing adversity (Snodgrass et al., 2019). While the chapters in this collection focused on positive psychological impact of games, this new research suggests that engaging in virtual worlds as a meaningful and recreational activity may also positively impact our well-being on the biological and chemical level.

Taken together, we hope that the essays contained within this book are just one of many steps toward shifting the perception of video games away from "How are they hurting us?" and toward "How are they helping us?" To change the focus from whether or not video games are making a generation of players violent, aggressive, and anti-social to determining how and why video games can be used for psychological growth, as tools to help cope with depression, anxiety, and stress by fostering persistence, self-care, and resilience. Building on the work discussed here, we hope to continue to explore how video games can foster psychological well-being and help us live happier, more satisfied lives.

References

Bowman, N. D., Kowert, R., & Ferguson, C. J. (2015). The impact of video game play on human (and orc) creativity. In G. Green & J. C. Kaufman (Eds.), *Video games and creativity* (pp. 39–60). San Diego, CA: Academic Press.

Brown, K. W., & Ryan, R. M. (2003). The benefits of being present: Mindfulness and its role in psychological well-being. *Journal of Personality and Social Psychology, 84*(4), 822–848.

Choi, B., & Baek, Y. (2011). Exploring factors of media characteristic influencing flow in learning through virtual worlds. *Computers & Education, 57*(4), 2382–2394.

Csikszentmihalyi, M. (1975). *Beyond boredom and anxiety.* San Francisco: Jossey-Bass.

Csikszentmihalyi, M. (1991). *Flow: The psychology of optimal experience.* New York: Harper Perennial.

Hamari, J., Shernoff, D. J., Rowe, E., Coller, B., Asbell-Clarke, J., & Edwards, T. (2016). Challenging games help students learn: An empirical study on engagement, flow and immersion in game-based learning. *Computers in Human Behavior, 54,* 170–179.

Hickson, J., Housley, W. F., & Boyle, C. (1988). The relationship of locus of control, age, and sex to life satisfaction and death anxiety in older persons. *The International Journal of Aging and Human Development, 26*(3), 191–199.

Huebner, E. S. (1991). Correlates of life satisfaction in children. *School Psychology Quarterly, 6*(2), 103.

Huebner, E. S., Ash, C., & Laughlin, J. E. (2001). Life experiences, locus of control, and school satisfaction in adolescence. *Social Indicators Research, 55*(2), 167–183.

Kiili, K. (2005). Digital game-based learning: Towards an experiential gaming model. *The Internet and Higher Education, 8*(1), 13–24.

Kowert, R., Festl, R., & Quandt, T. (2014). Unpopular, overweight, and socially inept: Reconsidering the stereotype of online gamers. *Cyberpsychology, Behavior, & Social Networking, 17*(3), 141–146. https://doi.org/10.1089/cyber.2013.0118.

Kowert, R., Griffiths, M., & Oldmeadow, J. A. (2012). Geek or Chic? Emerging stereotypes of online gamers. *Bulletin of Science, Technology & Society, 32*(6), 471–479. https://doi.org/10.1177/0270467612469078.

Mischel, W., Zeiss, R., & Zeiss, A. (1974). Internal-external control and persistence: Validation and implications of the Stanford preschool internal-external scale. *Journal of Personality and Social Psychology, 29*(2), 265.

Olson, C. K. (2015). Are electronic games health hazards or health promoters? In R. Kowert & T. Quandt (Eds.), *The video game debate* (pp. 39–53). New York, NY: Routledge.

Palmore, E., & Luikart, C. (1972). Health and social factors related to life satisfaction. *Journal of Health and Social Behavior, 13*(1), 68–80.

Rossin, D., Ro, Y. K., Klein, B. D., & Guo, Y. M. (2009). The effects of flow on learning outcomes in an online information management course. *Journal of Information Systems Education, 20*(1), 87–98.

Sliwinski, J., Katsikitis, M., & Jones, C. M. (2015, September). Mindful gaming: How digital games can improve mindfulness. In *IFIP Conference on Human-Computer Interaction* (pp. 167–184). Cham: Springer.

Snodgrass, J. G., Lacy, M. G., Francois, D. H. J., Polzer, E. R., Else, R. J., Arevalo, J. M. G., & Cole, S. W. (2019). Positive mental well-being and immune transcriptional profiles in highly involved video game player. *Brain, Behavior, and Immunity* (Published online ahead of print). https://doi.org/10.1016/j.bbi.2019.07.035.

Webster, J., Trevino, L. K., & Ryan, L. (1993). The dimensionality and correlates of flow in human-computer interaction. *Computers in Human Behavior, 9*, 411–426.

Index

A
avatar, 8, 49, 50, 52–57, 59–61, 100, 131–136, 161

C
cognitive dissonance, 114–118, 120

E
effectance, 5
eudaimonic well-being, 2, 6, 7, 9–11, 14, 15

F
feedback, 8, 67–69, 72, 74, 75, 100, 101, 118, 149, 161
flow, 5, 6, 14, 42, 90, 98–101, 103, 113, 132, 133, 160, 161

G
goal setting, 69, 70
growth mindset, 67, 70, 72–74, 160, 161

H
hedonic well-being, 2–6, 9, 14, 15

I
identity, 50–56, 60, 93, 119, 126, 128, 130, 149
identity crisis, 51
Interpersonal theory of personality development, 25
intrinsic motivators, 120

L
learning orientation, 69, 70, 74
loneliness, 12, 14, 57, 90

M
meaningful entertainment, 7, 10

R. Kowert (ed.), *Video Games and Well-being*,
Palgrave Studies in Cyberpsychology,
https://doi.org/10.1007/978-3-030-32770-5

mindfulness, 90, 93, 98, 99, 101–103, 160, 161
mood repair, 4
motivation, 3, 5, 9, 12, 24, 25, 67, 91, 92, 99, 111, 113, 114, 117, 119, 120, 162

N
narrative, 32, 33, 42, 51, 111, 127, 128, 130, 131, 147, 149, 151–154, 160, 161

P
positive psychology, 78–82, 89, 90
posttraumatic effects, 148, 154
posttraumatic growth, 151, 152, 154
posttraumatic stress disorder (PTSD), 142, 143, 146–150
psychological growth, 118, 160, 162

R
resilience, 78, 80–82, 84, 88, 127, 128, 142, 143, 148–153, 160–162
Role-Playing Games (RPG), 3, 12, 82, 88, 127, 129, 131–134, 136, 143

S
Self-Determination Theory (SDT), 7, 8, 11, 14
Self-Discrepancy Theory, 52
social capital, 11–15, 92
social learning theory, 52, 54
social support, 12, 149, 151, 153, 154
social well-being, 2, 11–15, 39, 126, 159
subjective well-being (SWB), 29, 31, 80, 81, 88

T
the Hero's Journey (tHJ), 127–131, 134–137, 161
trauma, 33, 39, 81, 142, 143, 146–149, 151, 152, 154

V
video games, 2, 10, 24, 27, 28, 32–34, 38–40, 43, 45, 50, 52–56, 60, 66–68, 70–72, 74, 78, 82, 84, 87, 89–93, 98–103, 110, 112, 113, 115, 121, 126–129, 133–136, 142, 144, 147, 154, 159–163
vulnerability, 56, 142, 143, 148–150, 153

W
well-being, 2–11, 13–15, 39, 78, 79, 90, 93, 98, 103, 126, 127, 131, 133, 136, 159–163